Essential Medical Biochemistry and Metabolic Disease

Vijay Yanamadala

Essential Medical Biochemistry and Metabolic Disease

A Pocket Guide for Medical Students and Residents

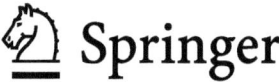

Vijay Yanamadala
Neurosurgery
Hartford Healthcare
Westport, CT, USA

ISBN 978-3-031-59393-2   ISBN 978-3-031-59394-9 (eBook)
https://doi.org/10.1007/978-3-031-59394-9

© The Editor(s) (if applicable) and The Author(s), under exclusive license to Springer Nature Switzerland AG 2024

This work is subject to copyright. All rights are solely and exclusively licensed by the Publisher, whether the whole or part of the material is concerned, specifically the rights of translation, reprinting, reuse of illustrations, recitation, broadcasting, reproduction on microfilms or in any other physical way, and transmission or information storage and retrieval, electronic adaptation, computer software, or by similar or dissimilar methodology now known or hereafter developed.

The use of general descriptive names, registered names, trademarks, service marks, etc. in this publication does not imply, even in the absence of a specific statement, that such names are exempt from the relevant protective laws and regulations and therefore free for general use.

The publisher, the authors and the editors are safe to assume that the advice and information in this book are believed to be true and accurate at the date of publication. Neither the publisher nor the authors or the editors give a warranty, expressed or implied, with respect to the material contained herein or for any errors or omissions that may have been made. The publisher remains neutral with regard to jurisdictional claims in published maps and institutional affiliations.

This Springer imprint is published by the registered company Springer Nature Switzerland AG

The registered company address is: Gewerbestrasse 11, 6330 Cham, Switzerland

If disposing of this product, please recycle the paper.

To my wife Vidya, who every day inspires me to be the best physician I can be for my patients and the best father I can be for our son.

Foreword

Back in the bad old days, biochemistry seemed like a tedious litany of metabolic pathways—relevant to clinical practice chiefly as a hurdle and rite of passage in medical school. You slogged through a massive tome (costing a significant fraction of your monthly living expenses), hopefully extracting the essentials that would get you through the exams. A year and a half later, you fell into the time-honored tradition of shelling out an additional smaller bundle to get the biochemistry review book that would help you get through the board exam. And then you promptly forgot 90% of it.

Fast forward to the brave new world of genomics and proteomics, a deluge of sequences and gel bands that allow the modeling of whole systems… and bring us to the brink of a whole new "omics"—metabolomics. Suddenly, the salient features of glycolysis have ramifications for cancer biology (Warburg effect, anyone?), mitochondrial dysfunction lies at the heart of myriad diseases, and we increasingly have the capacity to design small-molecule targets for a host of those previously esoteric biochemical pathways. Intermediary metabolism (AKA: biochemistry) has become relevant not only as a basic foundational building block in medical education but stands to provide some real therapeutic breakthroughs.

So you need to understand this stuff… just preferably without spending a fortune or getting bogged down in the arcane details. With all the other material you have got to master in med school, the more focused, organized, and relevant you can get biochemistry the first time, the better. Moreover, if it is accessible and understandable and pithy, you will come back to it again and again, like visiting an old friend.

Simply put, Vijay's Underground Guide to Medical Biochemistry and Metabolic Disease is what you need and truly all you need to prime your biochemistry pump… and provide the fundamental framework for med school, the boards… and beyond. Does it hold every detail? No. If you buy it and don't read it, will you pass the exam? No. Does it hold all the secrets of the universe? Not really. However, what it will do is provide the essentials in a crisp and elegant fashion, organize your thinking, and reduce your anxieties. I know this first hand because the students we have taught swear by it, and they did great in the course… and beyond.

Enjoy.

Richard N. Mitchell, MD, PhD
Harvard-MIT Division of Health Sciences and Technology
Lawrence J. Henderson Associate Professor of Pathology
Harvard Medical School
Boston, MA, USA

Preface

The purpose of this book is to efficiently provide students with the essentials of medical biochemistry that every medical student should know. Having served as instructor for the biochemistry course at Harvard Medical School in the Division of Health Sciences and Technology (HST) for 3 years, I came to realize that no current textbook delivers this material efficiently. With the limited time and ever-increasing amount of information out there, I hope this book will provide everything you need to know and nothing more.

There are three strategies to approaching anything in medical school. The first is to see the amount of material you have, be overwhelmed, and cover only a portion of what you need to know. The second is to spend countless days and nights poring through everything you've been given and memorize it down to the last detail. The third is to really understand why you are learning what you are learning so that you can really remember those details well into the future when you will use them. This third strategy is clearly the ideal one but is difficult to accomplish because we don't intrinsically know what the key concepts are before we begin. That's where this book is designed to help you. I have tried to emphasize key points so that you can develop that understanding of what is important and what isn't—and focus only on what is!

In using this book, your goal should really be twofold: (1) to understand the points of a metabolic pathway that contribute to disease pathogenesis and (2) to understand the points of those pathways that are therapeutically targeted and potentially targetable in the future. When you look at every pathway with these two goals in mind, it really comes alive and bears meaning that you might not have appreciated before. The importance of biochemistry within medicine is unquestionably growing, with new discoveries in all aspects of metabolism, from new work on the Warburg effect in carbohydrate metabolism, expanding discoveries on the pharmacology of eicosanoids and cholesterol in the realm of lipid metabolism, and the continuing investigation of proteasome inhibitors and nucleotide metabolism inhibitors as chemotherapeutics within the realms of amino acid and nucleotide metabolism, respectively. Understanding biochemistry will be central to taking care of patients and making new discoveries in medicine.

Most of the material in this book was written when I first taught HST biochemistry and was primarily designed to be review notes for the students. My students were so happy with my notes that they bound a copy of my notes into a book that they gifted me. They called it "Vijay's Underground Guide to Biochemistry," which is where the title of this book originated. Since that time, numerous people have encouraged me to turn this material into a book so that more people could benefit from it. It is my sincere hope that in finally putting this book together, I have provided a useful service to fellow medical students throughout the country.

In making this book possible, a number of people helped me tremendously. My first class of students in 2008 inspired me to write the original notes and encouraged me to compile them into this book. Dr. Richard N. Mitchell, the Associate Master of Health Sciences and Technology, and Dr. Charles N. Serhan, Professor of Anesthesiology and Biochemistry at Harvard Medical School, gave me invaluable advice throughout this process. I have to thank my parents and sister who helped me put the original book together more than a decade ago. And most importantly, I have to thank my wife who inspired me to finally publish this book with Springer Nature, along with the support of my father-in-law and mother-in-law, without which I could never have put this final version together.

With all my best, Vijay Yanamadala

Vijay Yanamadala, MD, MBA, FAANS, FCNS
Hartford Healthcare
Quinnipiac University Frank H. Netter School of Medicine
Sword Health
Westport, CT, USA

Contents

1 Carbohydrate Metabolism 1
   Pyruvate Metabolism 9
   Pyruvate Dehydrogenase...................... 10
      Succinate Thiokinase 12
      α-Ketoglutarate Dehydrogenase Complex 12
   Oxidative Phosphorylation 12
   Poisons of Oxidative Phosphorylation 13
   The Mitochondrial Shuttles of Carbohydrate
   Metabolism 14
   Glycogen................................... 16
      Glycogen Synthesis....................... 16
      Glycogenolysis 19
   The Glycogen Storage Disorders (GSDs).......... 21
   Gluconeogenesis............................. 22
      Conversion of Pyruvate to Phosphoenolpyruvate... 22
      Conversion of Fructose-1,6-Bisphosphate
      to Fructose-6-Phosphate 24
      Conversion of Glucose-6-Phosphate to Glucose.... 24
   The Cori Cycle 24
   Hexose Monophosphate Shunt (Pentose
   Phosphate Pathway) 25
   Insulin and Glucagon: Regulation of
   Glucose Metabolism 27
      Diseases................................ 28
   Fructose Metabolism......................... 29

The Sorbitol Pathway	31
Galactose Metabolism	31
Biochemical Changes During Exercise	32
Important Diseases of Carbohydrate Metabolism	33
Major Metabolic Diseases	33
Some Important Enzyme Deficiencies in Carbohydrate Metabolism	34

2   Lipid Metabolism

Lipid Metabolism	35
Biologically Important Lipids	35
Essential Fatty Acids	36
Harmful Fats	37
Simple Fatty Acids and Nutrition	37
Oxidation of Fatty Acids	42
Transport into the Mitochondrion: The Carnitine Shuttle	42
β-Oxidation	44
Energy Accounting	46
Oxidation of Unsaturated Fatty Acids	47
Peroxisomal Fatty Acid Metabolism	47
Ketone Body Formation	48
Lipogenesis (Fatty Acid Synthesis)	51
Fatty Acid Elongation	53
Synthesis of Monounsaturated and Polyunsaturated Fatty Acids	54
Regulation of Fatty Acid Synthesis	54
Insulin in Fatty Acid Metabolism	54
Comparing and Contrasting Fatty Acid Synthesis and Oxidation	55
Metabolism of Glycerolipids	56
Metabolism of Sphingolipids	57
The Sphingolipidoses and Sulfatidoses	58
Eicosanoids	62
Essential Differences Among the Eicosanoid Families	67
Metabolic Changes During Fasting	68
Cholesterol	69

Cholesterol Biosynthesis.	70
Regulation of HMG-CoA Reductase	72
Lipid Transport	72
Apolipoproteins.	73
Chylomicrons	73
Summary of Chylomicrons	74
VLDL, IDL, and LDL.	75
VLDL Summary	77
LDL Summary	77
HDL and Reverse Cholesterol Transport	77
HDL Summary	79
Other Lipoproteins of Note.	79
Disorders of Lipid Transport.	79
Lipid-Lowering Drugs	82
Clinical Aspects of Cholesterol Homeostasis	83
A Model of Atherogenesis	83
Cholesterol Metabolism	84
Bile Acids	84
Steroids	84
Congenital Adrenal Hyperplasia.	87
Androgens.	88
Female Sex Hormones	88
Vitamin D	88
Important Diseases of Lipid Metabolism	89
Major Metabolic Diseases.	89
Disorders of Lipid Transport (Table 2.4)	90
Some Important Enzyme Deficiencies in Carbohydrate Metabolism.	90
3 Amino Acid Metabolism.	**91**
Biologically Important Amino Acids	91
Overview of Amino Acid Metabolism	93
Biosynthesis of the Nutritionally Nonessential Amino Acids	93
Important Amino Acid Derivatives	100
The Essence of Protein Synthesis	102
Protein Degradation	103

Amino Acid Degradation 105
The Urea Cycle 106
　Regulation of the Urea Cycle 108
　Hepatic Encephalopathy 109
Ammonia Transport: The Glutamine Cycle 111
The Alanine Cycle 112
Catabolism of the Carbon Skeletons 113
Insulin and Glucagon in Amino Acid Metabolism 118
Porphyrin Synthesis and the Porphyrias 118
Hemoglobin 121
Porphyrin Degradation 122
Important Diseases of Amino Acid Metabolism 122
　Major Metabolic Diseases 122
　Some Important Enzyme Deficiencies
　in Amino Acid Metabolism 122

4 Nucleotide Metabolism 125
Biologically Important Nucleotides 125
Purine Nucleotide Biosynthesis 127
Regulation of De Novo Purine Biosynthesis 130
Chemotherapeutic Agents that Block Purine
Synthesis Enzymes 131
Purine Salvage 131
Synthesis of Deoxyribonucleotides 133
Purine Degradation: The Production of Uric Acid 134
Urate Pools 136
Causes of Hyperuricemia 136
Pathophysiology and Clinical
Manifestations of Gout 137
Treatment 137
Pyrimidine Biosynthesis 138
Regulation of Pyrimidine Biosynthesis 140
Chemotherapeutic Agents that Block
Pyrimidine Synthesis Enzymes 141
Pyrimidine Salvage 141
Pyrimidine Degradation 142
Rational Drug Design 142

Important Diseases of Nucleotide Metabolism....... 143
Major Metabolic Diseases..................... 143
Some Important Enzyme Deficiencies
in Carbohydrate Metabolism................... 143

5 **Vitamins**.................................... 145
$NAD^+/NADH$ and $FAD/FADH_2$:
The Biological REDOX Reagents 149
A Quick Review of REDOX Chemistry 149
Coupling Redox Reactions: The Importance
of Energetic Matching........................ 150
$NAD^+/NADH$ 151
$FAD/FADH_2$ Reductions..................... 151
Pyridoxine, Pyridoxal, and Pyridoxamine:
The Chemistry of Vitamin B_6 152
Pyridoxal Phosphate (PLP):
Chemical Reactivity 152
Folic Acid and Vitamin B12:
One Carbon Chemistry 155

Index 157

About the Author

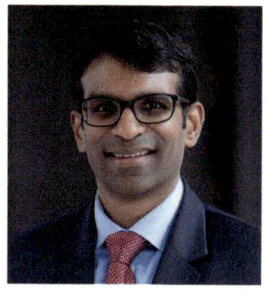

Vijay Yanamadala, MD, MBA, FAANS, FCNS is a board-certified neurosurgeon who specializes in the treatment of spinal disorders. He completed his undergraduate studies at Harvard University, where he studied biochemistry. He also completed a Master's Degree in Organic Chemistry at Harvard University, prior to earning his MD at Harvard Medical School. He completed his residency in neurological surgery at Massachusetts General Hospital.

He is currently an Associate Professor of Surgery (Neurosurgery) at the Quinnipiac University Frank H. Netter School of Medicine and serves as the System Medical Director of Spine Quality at Hartford Healthcare, the largest healthcare system in the state of Connecticut. He has extensive teaching experience, particularly in medical biochemistry.

In his clinical practice, he treats medical conditions including scoliosis, spine trauma, spinal vascular diseases, and spinal deformities. He has published over 80 scientific papers and received numerous awards on the safe and effective treatment of complex spinal conditions through advanced and innovative techniques paired with the use of multidisciplinary teams. Much of his work has centered on better coordination of musculoskeletal care and the avoidance of procedures and surgeries through care integration.

He is also a pioneering surgeon who was among the first surgeons in the tristate area and New England to offer awake spinal fusion surgery. He was also the second surgeon in the world to offer patient-specific spine fusion surgery. He has done international spine surgery missions in Kenya, India, Mongolia, and Sri Lanka, performing countless free surgeries during these trips. He is certified by the Safety in Spine Surgery Project (S3P) and is a member of the American Association of Neurological Surgeons, Congress of Neurological Surgeons, North American Spine Society, and the Scoliosis Research Society.

He also serves as Chief Medical Officer for Sword Health, the leading innovator for artificial intelligence in the healthcare sector.

Carbohydrate Metabolism

1

Biologically Important Monosaccharides are present naturally as D-isomers. Monosaccharides are divided into two major categories: **aldoses** and **ketoses**, depending on the oxidation state of the carbonyl carbon. Glucose represents the most important aldose, while fructose represents the most important aldose. Sugars are traditionally represented in three major forms: (1) acyclically as Fisher projections; (2) cyclically as Haworth projections; (3) cyclically in conformational form. Glucose is shown in these three forms in Fig. 1.1.

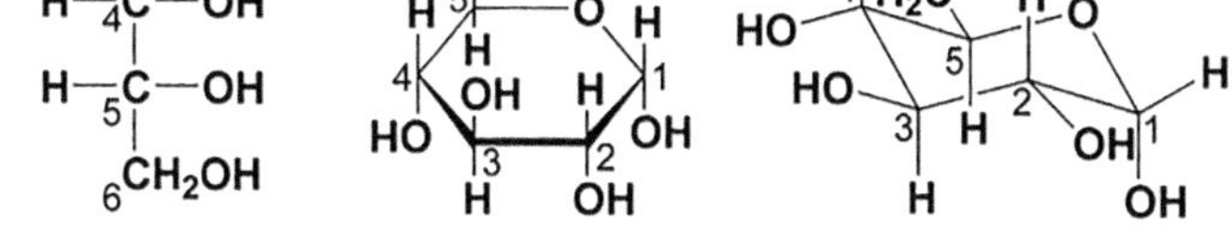

Fig. 1.1 D-glucose in its (**a**) Fischer projection, (**b**) Hayworth projection, and (**c**) chair configuration

© The Author(s), under exclusive license to Springer Nature Switzerland AG 2024
V. Yanamadala, *Essential Medical Biochemistry and Metabolic Disease*, https://doi.org/10.1007/978-3-031-59394-9_1

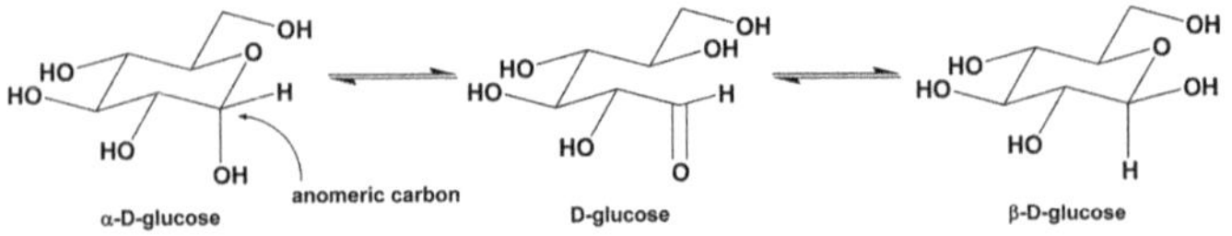

Fig. 1.2 Glucose represented in its common cyclical forms

Glucose is the most important monosaccharide, serving as the major metabolic fuel and the common precursor to all other monosaccharides and polysaccharides synthesized in the body. It is naturally present in three major forms, shown in Fig. 1.2. These are biologically relevant because particular catabolic and anabolic reactions use these conformers selectively. Many other cyclic and acyclic forms exist, but these are not particularly important. Notice in the acyclic form, the carbon 1 is an aldehyde. This is why glucose is categorized as an aldose.

β-D-glucose (β-D-glucopyranose) is the predominant form physiologically, although α-D-glucose (α-D-glucopyranose) is also found in substantial concentrations. The acyclic form is relatively sparse. The anomeric carbon is the carbon at which stereochemistry determines the α or β designation. The alpha carbon is the carbon whose stereochemistry determines the overall stereochemical designation of the molecule. D-glucose is R at the alpha carbon, while L-glucose is S at the alpha carbon. *The d and l designation have nothing to do with rotation of plane-polarized light, an unfortunate relic of biochemistry past.*

Polymers of glucose include glycogen, starch, and cellulose. Glycogen and starch are polymers of α-D-glucose and are thus metabolizable by the human body. Conversely, cellulose is a polymer of β-D-glucose and is thus non-metabolizable by the human body. It is the major dietary fiber.

Other hexoses include **fructose**, an isomer of glucose that is a ketose. Fructose is essentially glucose, in which carbon 1 is reduced to an alcohol and carbon 2 is oxidized to a ketone, hence its categorization as a ketose. This structure is shown in Fig. 1.3.

An important polymer of fructose is inulin, which is not digested in the intestine to oligosaccharides.

1 Carbohydrate Metabolism

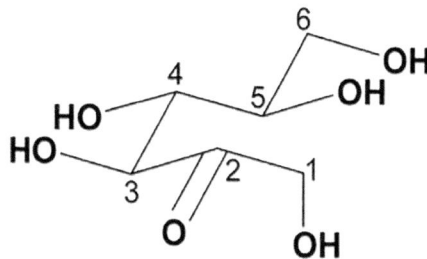

Fig. 1.3 Fructose

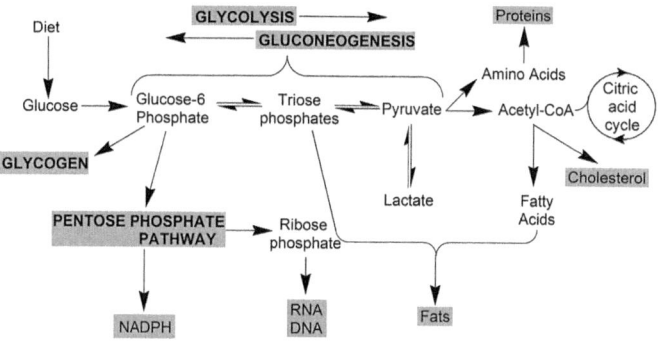

Fig. 1.4 Overview of carbohydrate metabolism

Galactose is an isomer (epimer) of glucose in which carbon 4 has the opposite stereochemistry. Galactose and glucose are interconverted in the body by a mechanism to be described subsequently.

Carbohydrate metabolism is centered around glycolysis, the major pathway by which glucose is utilized. An overview of the major aspects of carbohydrate metabolism are presented in Fig. 1.4.

Of course, the first step in carbohydrate metabolism, which is largely ignored, is digestion of dietary carbohydrates and uptake of monosaccharides. Digestion is generally taught in gastrointestinal pathophysiology courses and is thus only cursorily covered here. Briefly, uptake of glucose by enterocytes is mediated by the

Na$^+$-glucose cotransporter (**SGLT1**). Intracellular Na$^+$ concentrations are kept low by the action of the Na$^+$/K$^+$-ATPase, and it is this Na$^+$ gradient that drives the cotransport of Na$^+$ and glucose. Hence, transport of glucose into enterocytes is energy dependent.

The GLUT family of hexose transporters allow passive diffusion of glucose down its concentration gradient.

- **GLUT2** is a low-affinity transporter that allows for transport of glucose at high concentrations. It is present on the basolateral membrane of enterocytes and allows the glucose that was taken up by SGLT1 to diffuse into the interstitial fluid and ultimately the blood. GLUT2 is also present in the liver and pancreas, where it predominantly allows influx during states of high blood glucose to induce glycogen synthesis and insulin release, respectively, in these two tissues.
- **GLUT1** is constitutively expressed in the brain, erythrocytes, and other cells and allows for constitutive uptake of glucose in these cells. *Hence, in diabetic hyperglycemic states, high concentrations of glucose flood neurons and erythrocytes, damaging these cells and leading to diabetic neuropathy and erythrocyte dysfunction, respectively.*
- **GLUT4** is the insulin sensitive glucose transporter that is present in skeletal muscle and adipose tissue. GLUT4 is generally sequestered in cytosolic vessels. Insulin signaling activates PI3K, which causes vesicles containing GLUT4 to fuse with the plasma membrane, allowing for increased glucose transport. These tissues predominantly take up glucose when insulin levels are high, but alternative pathways such as activation of AMPK may also induce GLUT4 translocation to the plasma membrane.
- **GLUT5** is a fructose transporter.

Glycolysis is classically characterized by ten enzymatic reactions that yield two molecules of pyruvate from each molecule of glucose, along with a net two ATP and two NADH. The steps of glycolysis are shown in Fig. 1.5.

1 Carbohydrate Metabolism

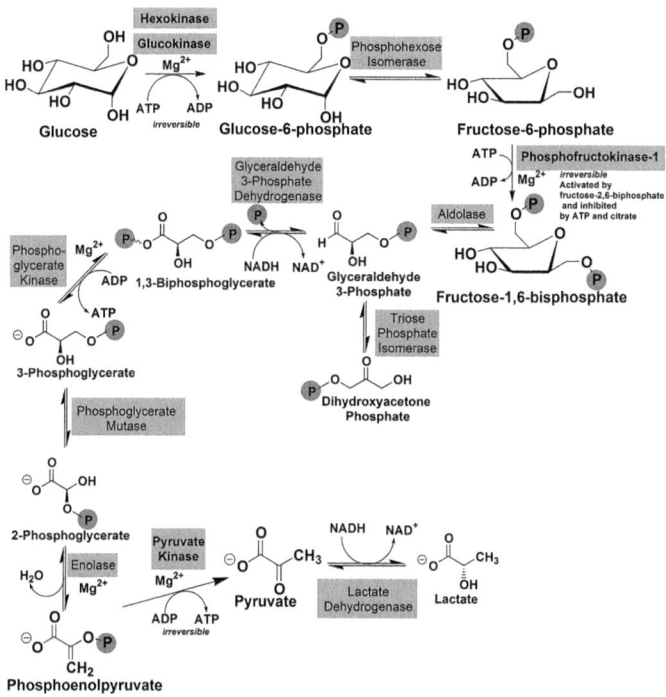

Fig. 1.5 Glycolysis. Key enzymes to know are those that catalyze the irreversible steps, hexokinase (glucokinase), phosphofructokinase-1, and pyruvate kinase. Phosphofructokinase-1 is the rate limiting step in glycolysis and is the most regulated step

Step 1: Phosphorylation of Glucose

This step, shown in more detail in Fig. 1.6, is *irreversible* and is carried out either by hexokinase or glucokinase. Hexokinase is a constitutively active enzyme that has a small Km and is present in every cell of the body. It serves to trap glucose in the cell as glucose-6-phosphate (glucose-6-phosphate cannot exit the cell) and also acts to funnel glucose into the cell by keeping concentrations of free glucose low. It is thus a *flux generating* reaction. Glucokinase is present in the **liver** and **pancreas** and

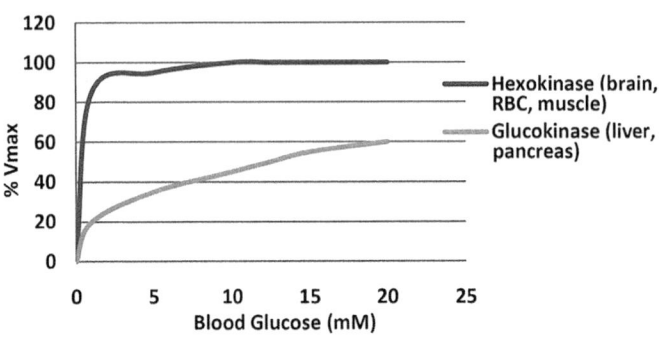

Fig. 1.6 The enzyme kinetics of hexokinase and glucokinase

has a high Km, which means that it predominantly functions at high concentrations of glucose. The low Km of hexokinase causes it to become saturated with glucose at low concentrations, without substantial change in response to varying concentrations of glucose. *Additionally, hexokinase, but not glucokinase, is inhibited by its product, glucose-6-phosphate.* The high Km of glucokinase, on the other hand, means that it can modulate the rate of glucose phosphorylation over the physiological range. Its rate of glucose phosphorylation substantially increases when glucose concentrations increase. *One molecule of ATP is expended in this step.* The kinetics of this step are shown in Fig. 1.7.

Step 2: Isomerization of Glucose-6-Phosphate to Fructose-6-Phosphate

Phosphohexose isomerase catalyzes this step.

Step 3: Phosphorylation of Fructose-6-Phosphate

This is the rate determining step (RDS) of glycolysis and is the most regulated step. *Understanding the details of this step is essential to understanding the regulation and dysregulation of glycolysis.* Fructose-6-phosphate is phosphorylated at the 1-position by **phosphofructokinase-1**. *This enzyme is negatively regulated by ATP and citrate, both markers of glycolysis end-products.* As you will see, the acetyl-CoA synthesized

1 Carbohydrate Metabolism

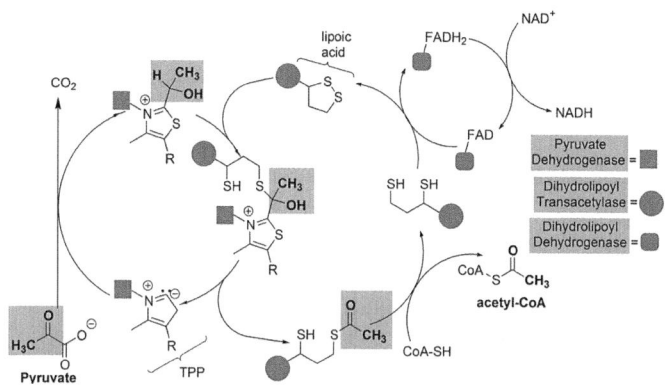

Fig. 1.7 Pyruvate is converted to acetyl-CoA and CO_2 by the pyruvate dehydrogenase complex, which consists of three enzymes, pyruvate dehydrogenase, dihydrolipoyl transacetylase, and dihydrolipoyl dehydrogenase. Pyruvate dehydrogenase uses thiamine and lipoic acid as co-factors, yielding acetyl-lipoic acid. Lipoic acid is then exchanged with coenzyme A to yield acetyl-CoA. The function of the other two enzymes is the regeneration of lipoic acid

at by pyruvate dehydrogenase is used to transform oxaloacetate to citrate as part of the tricarboxylic acid cycle. *Alternatively, it is activated by fructose-2,6-bisphosphate (F2,6BP) and AMP.* This is produced by the enzyme **phosphofructokinase-2/fructose-2,6-bisphosphatase**. This is a bifunctional enzyme that can phosphorylate fructose-6-phosphate using ATP to F2,6BP and dephosphorylate it back to fructose-6-phosphate by releasing inorganic phosphate. *Realize that this is not a reversible reaction. This is a bifunctional enzyme that catalyzes two irreversible reactions. One molecule of ATP is expended in this step.*

The kinase activity and phosphatase activity of PFK-2/F2,6BP are tightly regulated by insulin and glucagon signaling. Phosphorylation of this enzyme by PKA, as occurs with glucagon signaling, increases phosphatase activity and decreases kinase activity. Dephosphorylation of this enzyme, as occurs in the presence of insulin signaling, leads to increased kinase activity and decreased phosphatase activity.

Step 4: Reverse Aldol (Retroaldol) Cleavage

Aldolase performs the reverse aldol reaction yielding two triose molecules, dihydroxyacetone-1-phosphate (DHAP) and glyceraldehyde-1-phosphate (GAP) from fructose 1,6-bisphosphate. *Inherited aldolase A deficiency in erythrocytes causes hemolytic anemia because mature erythrocytes, which lack mitochondria, are completely dependent on glycolysis for ATP synthesis.*

Step 5: Isomerization of Dihydroxyacetone Phosphate to Glyceraldehyde Phosphate

The equilibrium between DHAP and GAP is favorable to DHAP, which is present at a concentration 20 times greater than that of GAP in the cytoplasm of a cell. However, GAP is required for the final production of pyruvate in glycolysis and is the active substrate for the next step of glycolysis. Thus, **triose phosphate isomerase** (TIM) is a necessary equilibrase which quickly reequilibrates the system so as to ensure a constant supply of GAP for the progress of glycolysis. TIM is one of the most efficient enzymes known—it is only limited by the rate of diffusion of its substrates!

Step 6: Generation of NADH through the Oxidative Phosphorylation of GAP

GAP is oxidatively phosphorylated to 1,3-bisphosphoglycerate by glyceraldehyde-1-phosphate dehydrogenase (GAPDH), in the process reducing one molecule of NAD^+ to NADH. Thus, per molecule of glucose, two molecules of NADH are produced during this step. Note that this step is critically dependent upon the presence of NAD^+, and in its absence, glycolysis comes to a halt. This is the purpose of lactate generation, as discussed below.

Step 7: Generation of ATP through the Dephosphorylation of 1,3-bisphosphoglycerate

Glycerate Kinase catalyzes the formation of ATP from ADP through the dephosphorylation of the carboxylic phosphate of 1,3BPG, yielding 3-phosphoglycerate. Importantly, in erythrocytes, an alternative pathway allows for the formation of

2,3-bisphosphoglycerate (2,3BPG), an important allosteric regulator of hemoglobin. 1,3BPG is isomerized to 2,3BPG by bisphosphoglycerate mutase, and 2,3BPG can then be metabolized to 3-phosphoglycerate by 2,3-bisphosphoglycerate phosphatase. This does not allow the formation of ATP, however.

Step 8: Isomerization of Phosphoglycerate

Phosphoglycerate mutase isomerizes 3-phosphoglycerate to 2-phosphoglycerate.

Step 9: Dehydration of 2-Phosphoglycerate

Enolase dehydrates 2-phosphoglycerate to produce 2-phosphoenolpyruvate.

Step 10: Generation of Pyruvate

Pyruvate Kinase produces ATP by dephosphorylating phosphoenolpyruvate, in the process yielding the final product of glycolysis, pyruvate. *Pyruvate kinase is activated by fructose-1,6-bisphosphate and inhibited by ATP and alanine*, once again carrying forth the notion of substrate activation and product inhibition for metabolic pathways. *Inherited pyruvate kinase deficiency in erythrocytes causes hemolytic anemia.*

Each NADH produced through glycolysis may yield either two or three ATP, depending on which *mitochondrial shuttle* is used to transmit its reducing equivalents to the mitochondrial matrix for oxidative phosphorylation. If the **glycerolphosphate shuttle** is used, each NADH will yield two ATP. If the **malate-aspartate shuttle (malate shuttle)** is used, each NADH will yield three ATP. The details of these shuttles will be discussed subsequently.

Pyruvate Metabolism

Pyruvate is a substrate for a number of reactions. In the average cell, pyruvate becomes the substrate for **pyruvate dehydrogenase**, a mitochondrial enzyme that decarboxylates pyruvate and produces acetyl-coenzyme A (acetyl-coA). The mechanism is discussed below. Under reducing conditions (such as hypoxia) or in cells that lack mitochondria (such as erythrocytes), pyruvate is reduced to lactate by **lactate dehydrogenase**. This expends NADH, thus making NAD^+ available for continued glycolysis. Thus, this expends all NADH produced in glycolysis, yielding a net of **two ATP** molecules per glucose molecule under these conditions (because there is no net NADH production). Alternatively, pyruvate can be converted to the amino acid alanine by **alanine aminotransferase** (ALT; also known as serum glutamate pyruvate transaminase, SGPT). There are many other reactions as well.

Pyruvate Dehydrogenase

Under oxidative conditions, pyruvate is readily taken up into mitochondria, where it is decarboxylated to acetyl-coenzyme A (acetyl-CoA) by pyruvate dehydrogenase in a complex reaction that requires five vitamin cofactors (thiamin as thiamine diphosphate, riboflavin as FAD, niacin as NAD^+, pantothenic acid in coenzyme A, and lipoic acid) and three minerals (Ca^{2+}, Mg^{2+}, and PO_4^{3-}). This is a complex reaction, as shown in Fig. 1.8, and is highly regulated by insulin and other metabolites, as shown in Fig. 1.9.

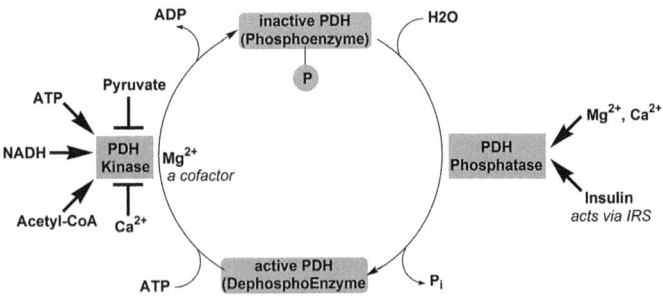

Fig. 1.8 Pyruvate dehydrogenase is a highly regulated enzyme. Both its endproducts, acetyl-CoA, NADH, and ATP, as well as insulin and cations, regulate its function, as depicted above. Arrows indicate activation, while dashes indicate inhibition

Pyruvate Dehydrogenase

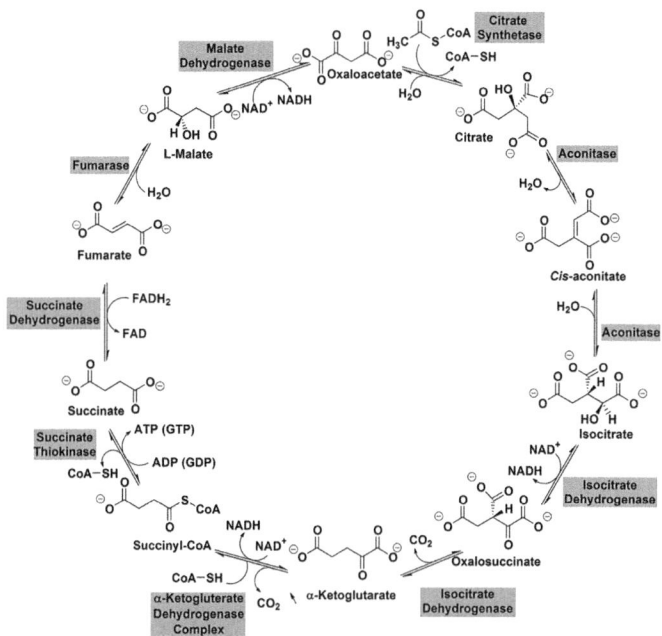

Fig. 1.9 The tricarboxylic acid cycle (Kreb cycle), through which acetyl-CoA is converted to CO_2 and three molecules of NADH, one molecule of $FADH_2$, and one molecule of ATP or GTP. The energy in NADH and $FADH_2$ is ultimately converted to ATP through oxidative phosphorylation. Importantly, the TCA serves as an entry point for a number of other intersecting metabolic pathways, as will be discussed in Chap. 3

Mutations in pyruvate dehydrogenase lead to congenital lactic acidosis. Arsenite and mercuric ions react with the thiol groups of lipoic acid and thus inhibit pyruvate dehydrogenase, as does a dietary deficiency of thiamin, also leading to lactic acidosis. Arsenic toxicity is characterized by vomiting, rice water stools, and garlic breath. Many alcoholics are thiamin-deficient (both because of a poor diet and also because alcohol inhibits thiamin absorption) and may develop potentially fatal pyruvic and lactic acidosis.

The ***Tricarboxylic Acid Cycle (TCA; Kreb's Cycle; Citric Acid Cycle)*** is an important **amphibolic** pathway (a pathway that serves both catabolic and anabolic purposes). Catabolically, it allows for the generation of ATP by the oxidative phosphorylation chain from acetyl-CoA produced by pyruvate dehydrogenase by producing NADH and $FADH_2$. Anabolically, it is important in gluconeogenesis, lipogenesis, and the interconversion of amino acids.

The enzymes of the TCA are found in the mitochondrial matrix.

Succinate Thiokinase

The liver and kidney (tissues capable of gluconeogenesis) contain two isoforms of succinate thiokinase, one that produces ATP from ADP (the isoform found in all tissues) and another that produces GTP from GDP. This isoform is important in these gluconeogenic tissues because GTP is essential for the function of phosphoenolpyruvate carboxykinase, an essential enzyme in gluconeogenesis.

Mnemonic **C**itrate **I**s **K**reb's **S**tarting **S**ubstrate **F**or **M**aking **O**xaloacetate (this gives you each of the intermediates in the TCA in order).

α-Ketoglutarate Dehydrogenase Complex

This enzyme complex is analogous to the pyruvate dehydrogenase complex and requires the same cofactors.

Oxidative Phosphorylation

The enzymes involved in oxidative phosphorylation are located within the inner mitochondrial membrane. Oxidative phosphorylation allows for the conversion of energy in the form of NADH and $FADH_2$ produced during the TCA and glycolysis into ATP. It is wholly dependent upon oxygen, which acts as the final electron acceptor in the chain. The major physiological function of molecular oxygen is to serve as the final electron acceptor during respiration. The **chemiosmotic theory** proposes that the proton gradient generated by the electron transport chain, shown below, is the driving force for ATP synthesis by the F0/F1 ATPase. Protons flow through the ATPase back into the mitochondrial matrix, and this causes the phosphorylation of ADP to ATP. ATP/ADP exchangers exist in the inner mitochondrial membrane to exchange ADP in the cytosol for ADP in the matrix. *The electrochemical gradient across the inner mitochondrial membrane favors the export of ATP (which is quadruply charged) and import of ADP (which is triply charged).* Hence the proton gradient not only functions to promote ATP synthesis but is also important for ATP export to the cytosol.

Importantly, within the electron transport chain, NADH enters at complex I while $FADH_2$ enters at complex II. Thus, NADH causes the translocation of approximately 3–4 more protons than $FADH_2$. This explains a fundamental and important difference between NADH and $FADH_2$ energetics: *NADH yields ~3 ATP per molecule, while $FADH_2$ yields ~2 ATP per molecule.*

Poisons of Oxidative Phosphorylation

Ionophores (uncouplers) permit the dissipation of the proton gradient and thus prevent ATP synthesis. **Dinitrophenol** is the classic uncoupler. Additionally, a physiological uncoupler, **thermogenin (UCP1)**, is present in brown fat and serves to generate heat by simply dissipating the energy stored within the proton gradient. It is the primary mechanism by which human infants maintain body temperature. **Aspirin** can also act as an uncoupler, which is why aspirin overdose can be associated with fevers!

Oligomycin directly inhibits the F0/F1 ATPase, thus preventing ATP synthesis. This is associated with an increased proton gradient across the inner mitochondrial membrane.

Rotenone, CN^- (cyanide), antimycin A, and CO (carbon monoxide) directly inhibit the various electron transport complexes and thus prevent the development of the proton gradient that is essential for ATP synthesis.

MELAS (mitochondrial encephalopathy, lactic acidosis, and stroke) is an inherited deficiency in complex I or complex IV. There are several other mitochondrial disorders that also involve mutations in the proteins of the respiratory chain, most of them with severe phenotypes.

The Mitochondrial Shuttles of Carbohydrate Metabolism

NADH produced during glycolysis must ultimately be oxidized in the mitochondria in order to yield ATP. However, the inner mitochondrial membrane is impermeable to both NAD^+ and NADH. Thus, two shuttles have been designed to transport the electrons from NADH into the mitochondria. These are the **glycerolphosphate shuttle** and the **malate-aspartate shuttle**.

The glycerolphosphate shuttle, shown in Fig. 1.10, allows for the production of ~2ATP per NADH produced during glycolysis. In the cytosol, glycerol-3-phosphate dehydrogenase reduces dihydroxyacetone phosphate (DHAP) produced by aldolase to glycerol-3-phosphate. This regenerates cytosolic NAD^+ for continued glycolysis. Glycerol-3-phosphate readily penetrates the outer mitochondrial membrane. A different isoform of glycerol-3-phosphate dehydrogenase then reoxidizes glycerol-3-phosphate back to DHAP, in the process reducing FAD to $FADH_2$. Hence, there is a net conversion of cytosolic NADH to mitochondrial $FADH_2$. Each molecule of $FADH_2$ then produces two molecules of ATP. Hence, tissues where this shuttle is present produce ~36 ATP from the metabolism of 1 glucose molecule (6 ATP from glycolysis; 6 ATP from pyruvate dehydrogenase generated NADH; 24 from the TCA). Unlike the malate shuttle which is found in all tissues, the glycerolphosphate shuttle is found in very few tissues, the brain being an important example. Teleologically, it is possible that the coexistence of two shuttles in the brain serves as a redundancy mechanism.

The malate shuttle, shown in Fig. 1.11, is a more complex shuttle that produces the net conversion of cytosolic NADH to mitochondrial NADH. Each molecule of NADH then produces

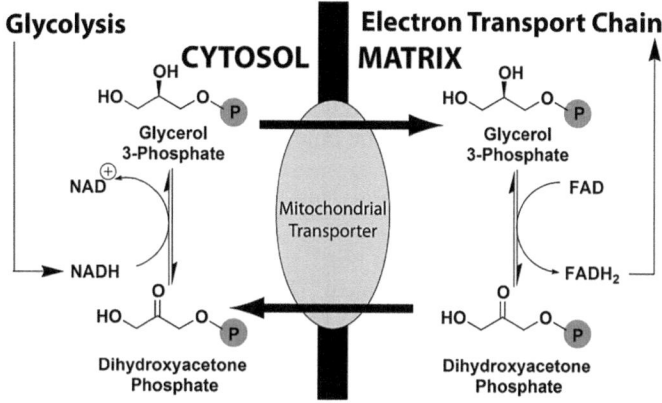

Fig. 1.10 The glycerol phosphate shuttle

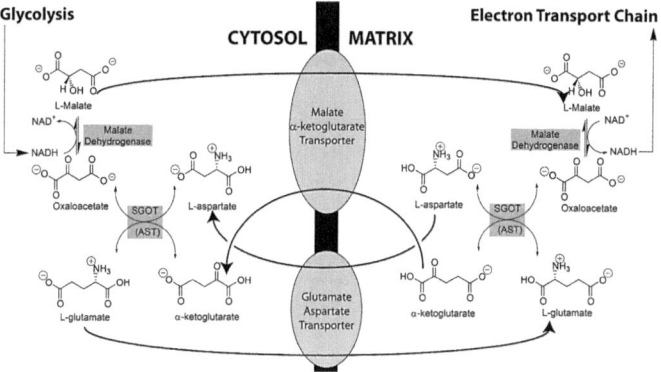

Fig. 1.11 The malate shuttle

three molecules of ATP. Hence, tissues where this shuttle is present produce ~**38 ATP** from the metabolism of 1 glucose molecule (8 ATP from glycolysis; 6 ATP from pyruvate dehydrogenase generated NADH; 24 from the TCA). The heart relies exclusively on the malate shuttle. All tissues possess the malate shuttle.

The creatine phosphate shuttle is important in muscle, especially during periods of high ATP production and low ATP usage. Creatine phosphate is an important cytosolic store of high-energy phosphate that can be readily converted to ATP as needed. Creatinine is a smaller molecule than ADP and is thus a less energetically costly storage form (adenosine has to be synthesized, as we will learn about in Chap. 4, in order to make ATP). Cytosolic creatine is transmitted into the mitochondrial matrix, where it is phosphorylated.

Glycogen

Glycogen is an important storage form of glucose. It is a branched polymer of α-D-glucose, consisting of both α1 → 4 and α1 → 6 linkages. These two linkages are shown in Fig. 1.12.

Branching is important because (1) it allows for more compact packing of glycogen and (2) allows for faster polymerization and depolymerization because only terminal monomers of glucose may be added or removed. Hence, branching allows for the existence of numerous terminal points for the addition or removal of glucose.

Glycogen Synthesis

An overview of glycogen synthesis is provided in Fig. 1.13. The first step of glycogen synthesis is priming. Glucose-6-phosphate is converted first to glucose-1-phosphate in a reversible reaction

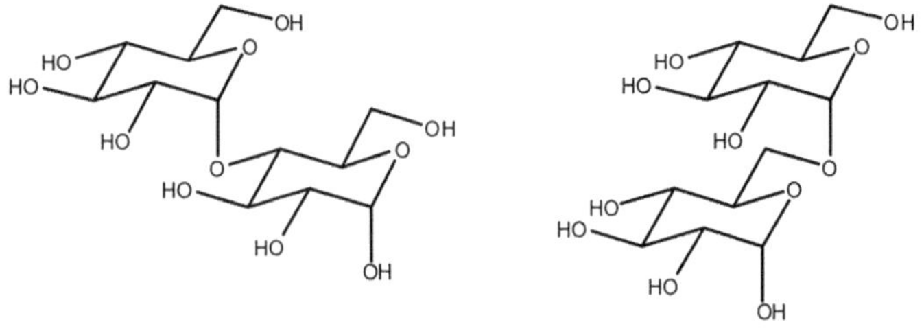

Fig. 1.12 Representations of glycogen linkages

Glycogen

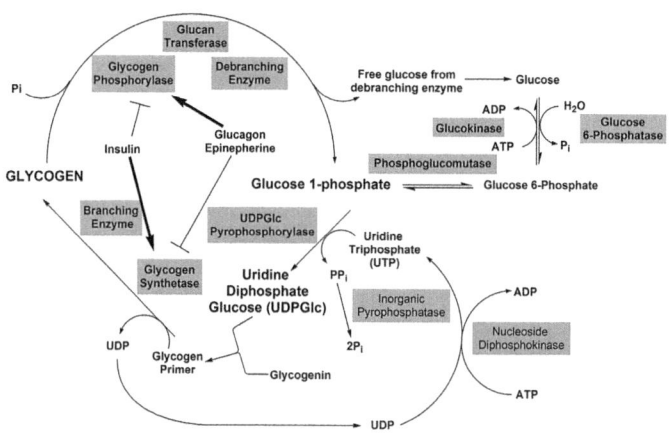

Fig. 1.13 Pathways of glycogen synthesis and glycogenolysis in the liver and their regulation. Arrows indicate activation, while dashes indicate inhibition

catalyzed by **phosphoglucomutase**. Glucose-1-phosphate is then converted to UDP-glucose with the expenditure of UTP. Notice here that UTP and glucose-6-phosphate are converted to UDP-glucose and pyrophosphate (PPi). The pyrophosphate is then hydrolyzed by **pyrophosphatase** to two phosphates, releasing ~5 kcal/mol of energy. *This is the driving force for the formation of UDP-glucose and hence glycogen itself. Remember that polymerization reactions are almost always endergonic because there is a reduction in entropy. Hence, hydrolysis of pyrophosphate provides a powerful driving force for glucose polymerization into glycogen.*

The second step is synthesis of the straight chain α1 → 4 chain. This is accomplished by glycogen synthase, which takes UDP-glucose as its substrate and adds it to a preformed glycogen chain, releasing UDP in the process. This UDP is then freed to reform UTP for continued production of UDP-glucose. This is shown in Fig. 1.14.

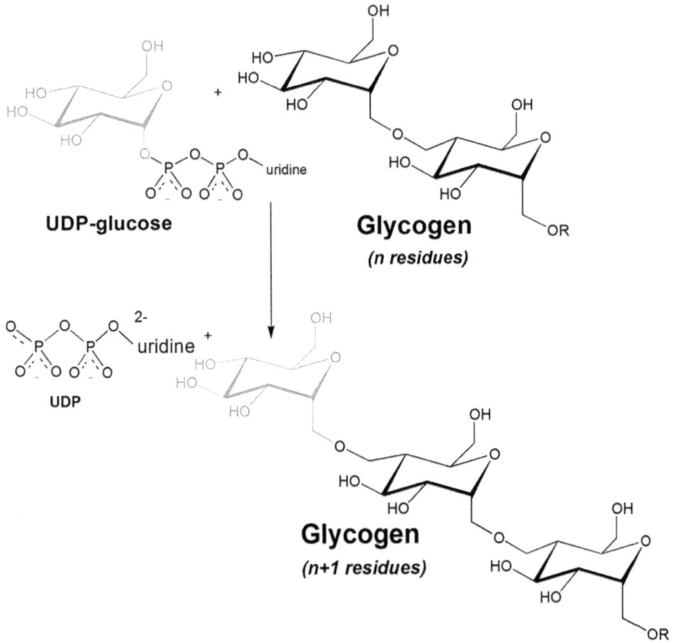

Fig. 1.14 Synthesis of the α1 → 4 linkage

Some essential points about glycogen synthase:

- It is the rate-limiting enzyme of glycogen synthesis.
- It is constitutively active.
- Its activity is upregulated by G6P and insulin signaling (which maintains it in a dephosphorylated state).
- It is inactivated by phosphorylation (therefore by PKA via glucagon and epinephrine signaling—both signal by activating the heterotrimeric G protein, Gαs, leading to cAMP production and PKA activation).

The third step in glycogen synthesis is branching. Once chain at least 11 residues, branching occurs: specifically, amylo-(1,4-1,6)-transglycosylase (the branching enzyme) removes a chain of 7

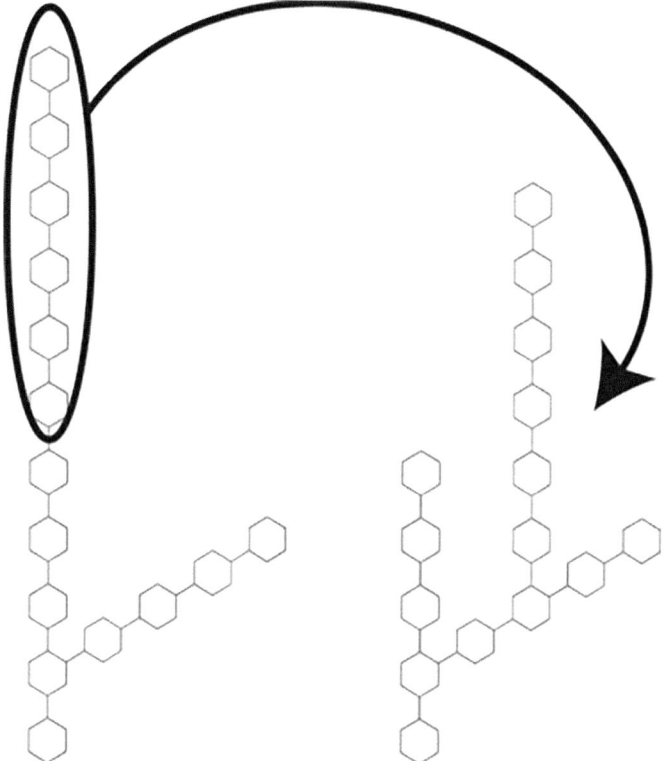

Fig. 1.15 The branching enzyme breaks α1 → 4 linkages and makes α1 → 6 linkages to create a branch point

glucoses and attaches it to another chain by an α1 → 6 glycosidic bond, as shown in Fig. 1.15.

Glycogenolysis

The first step of glycogenolysis is the breakdown of terminal glucose residues to glucose-1-phosphate by **glycogen phosphorylase**. This requires the addition of inorganic phosphate, and the driving force for this reaction is largely entropic.

Some essential points about glycogen phosphorylase:

- It is rate-limiting enzyme of glycogenolysis.
- It is inhibited by ATP, G6P, and insulin signaling (which leads to dephosphorylation).
- It is activated by phosphorylase kinase (therefore by glucagon, epinephrine, PKA, high Ca^{2+}).

The second step of glycogenolysis is debranching. Glycogen phosphorylase stops four residues from a branchpoint and is unable to proceed. At this point, glucotransferase relocates the terminal 3 glucose residues to a free C4 end, making a new α1 → 4 bond. Then, the α1 → 6 bond is broken by glucosidase (the debranching enzyme). This process is shown in Fig. 1.16.

Finally, free glucose-1-phosphate is converted to glucose-6-phosphate by phosphoglucomutase.

Glycogen synthesis is largely limited to the liver and muscle. The liver contains **glucose-6-phosphatase**, which is capable of hydrolyzing glucose-6-phosphate back to glucose, releasing inor-

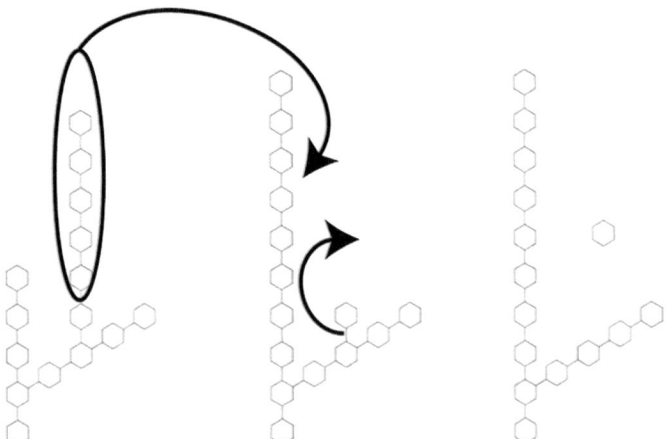

Fig. 1.16 Glucan transferase first transfers chains, leaving only the last glucose attached by the α1 → 6 linkage. The debranching enzyme then cleaves this α1 → 6 linkage to release free glucose

ganic phosphate. This free glucose can then diffuse out of hepatocytes into the bloodstream. Conversely, muscle does not have glucose-6-phosphatase. Because only free glucose can diffuse into and out of cells, muscle glycogen can never be converted to free glucose and thus glucose stored as muscle glycogen cannot be directly exported from the muscle. Importantly, this is correlated with a major functional distinction between hepatic glycogen and muscle glycogen. Hepatic glycogen functions to maintain blood glucose levels during fasting. Muscle glycogen largely serves as a readily mobilizable pool of glucose during periods of intense activity.

Liver glycogen maintains blood glucose concentrations during early stages of fasting. Liver glycogen is typically depleted within 12–18 h of fasting, although there is some variability. After this, the liver switches to gluconeogenesis, which is described below.

The Glycogen Storage Disorders (GSDs)

The glycogen storage disorders are a class of congenital disorders resulting from deficiencies (mutations) in various enzymes involved in glycogen synthesis or glycogenolysis. While there are numerous disorders, some key disorders with which you should be familiar are listed below.

Type 0: Glycogen synthase deficiency results in early death from hypoglycemia.

Type I (Von Gierke Disease): glucose-6-phosphatase deficiency results in hypoglycemia and lactic acidosis and ketoacidosis.

Type II (Pompe Disease): Lysosomal α-glucosidase deficiency results in death from heart failure, generally by age 2.

Type III (Forbes Disease): Debranching enzyme deficiency results in hypoglycemia and the accumulation of limit dextrins in the liver.

Type IV (Andersen Disease): Branching enzyme deficiency results in hepatosplenomegaly with death from heart or liver failure, generally by age 2.

Type V (McArdle Disease): Muscle phosphorylase deficiency results in poor exercise tolerance.

Type VI (Her Disease): Liver phosphorylase deficiency results in hepatomegaly with hypoglycemia.

Gluconeogenesis

Gluconeogenesis involves the generation of glucose from pyruvate. It is carried out by the liver and to some extent by the kidney. The three irreversible steps of glycolysis (glucokinase, phosphofructokinase-1, and pyruvate kinase) must be reversed by separate enzymes. All other steps are simply the reverse of glycolysis. A schematic of gluconeogenesis is provided in Fig. 1.17. A summary of the three irreversible steps is provided below.

Conversion of Pyruvate to Phosphoenolpyruvate

This is a complex reaction involving two enzymes. Pyruvate diffuses from the cytosol into the mitochondrial matrix. Here, **pyruvate carboxylase** carboxylates it to oxaloacetate. Oxaloacetate proceeds TCA to produce malate, which diffuses out of the mitochondrion into the cytosol. In the cytosol, malate is oxidized to oxaloacetate, generating NADH. Pyruvate carboxylase requires biotin and ATP and is ***activated by acetyl-CoA***. This makes metabolic sense, because the accumulation of acetyl-CoA implies that there is a rate of glycolysis that exceeds the cell's TCA cycle capacity.

Oxaloacetate is then phosphorylated and decarboxylated to phosphoenolpyruvate by **phosphoenolpyruvate carboxykinase**. ***This step requires GTP***. Remember that in gluconeogenic tissues, succinate thiokinase, and enzyme of the TCA, can produce GTP instead of ATP. This is an important link between the TCA and gluconeogenesis that serves to co-modulate the activities of the two processes.

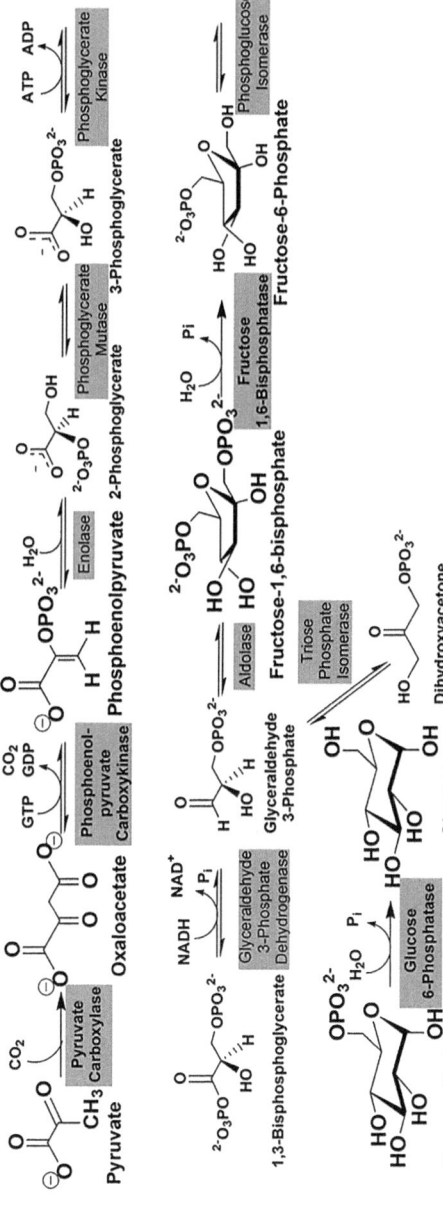

Fig. 1.17 Gluconeogenesis. The three key steps in gluconeogenesis that differ from glycolysis are (1) the conversion of pyruvate to phosphoenolpyruvate, (2) the conversion of fructose-1,6-bisphosphate to fructose-6-phosphate, and (3) the conversion of glucose-6-phosphate to glucose. Notice that these processes are the reverse of the three irreversible steps in glycolysis. Hence, they require unique enzymes, as discussed in the text. All other steps in gluconeogenesis are identical to their reverse steps in glycolysis

Conversion of Fructose-1,6-Bisphosphate to Fructose-6-Phosphate

This is achieved by **fructose-1,6-bisphosphatase**, which releases inorganic phosphate. Fructose-2,6-bisphophate (F2,6BP) is an important allosteric inhibitor of this enzyme. Remember that F2,6BP is also an allosteric activator of phosphofructokinase-1.

Conversion of Glucose-6-Phosphate to Glucose

This final step is achieved by **glucose-6-phosphatase**, releasing inorganic phosphate in the process.

Mnemonic **P**athways **P**roduce **F**resh **G**lucose (the four enzymes of gluconeogenesis that reverse the irreversible steps of glycolysis, in their order). ***These enzymes are present in the liver and kidney, as well as to some extent in the intestinal epithelium.*** Thus, these are the only tissues capable of gluconeogenesis.

The Cori Cycle

The Cori cycle is an important means by which lactate produced systemically is recycled to the liver to be converted back to pyruvate and eventually glucose via gluconeogenesis. Thus, this prevents lactate buildup, which can lead to lactic acidosis. This also allows for continued glycolysis in muscle during strenuous exercise by funneling the product, lactate. A summary is provided in Fig. 1.18.

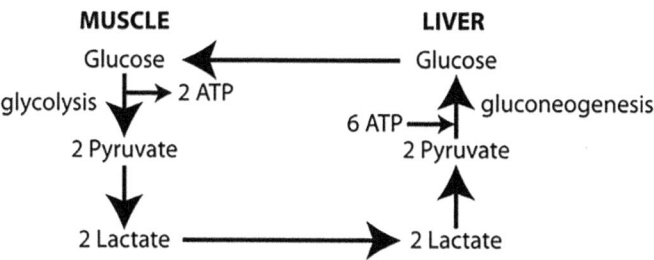

Fig. 1.18 The Cori cycle. Lactate produced in muscle through glycolysis is recycled through the bloodstream to the liver, where it is converted to glucose through gluconeogenesis

Hexose Monophosphate Shunt (Pentose Phosphate Pathway)

This pathway is an alternative sink for glucose-6-phosphate and is important for (1) the formation of **NADPH** that is utilized in anabolic processes such as fatty acid synthesis and steroid synthesis and (2) the synthesis of **ribose** used for nucleotide synthesis.

A diagram of the HMP Shunt is given in Fig. 1.19. Notice that glucose-6-phosphate is both the initial substrate and the final product of this shunt. The purpose of this shunt is to give access to all of the intermediate sugars for intermediary metabolism. Ultimately, glucose-6-phosphate can finally be utilized for glycolysis.

The HMP shunt is divided into two phases: the irreversible oxidative phase and the reversible non-oxidative phase. The oxidative phase produces NADPH and occurs in tissues where NADPH is essential including the liver (fatty acid synthesis), adipose tissue (fatty acid synthesis), adrenal cortex (steroid hormone synthesis), thyroid gland (thyroid hormone synthesis), erythrocytes (reduction of glutathione, an antioxidant), testis (steroid hormone synthesis), and neutrophils (oxidative burst). The non-oxidative phase allows for the formation of various metabolic trioses, tetroses, pentoses, and heptoses, the most important of which is ribose.

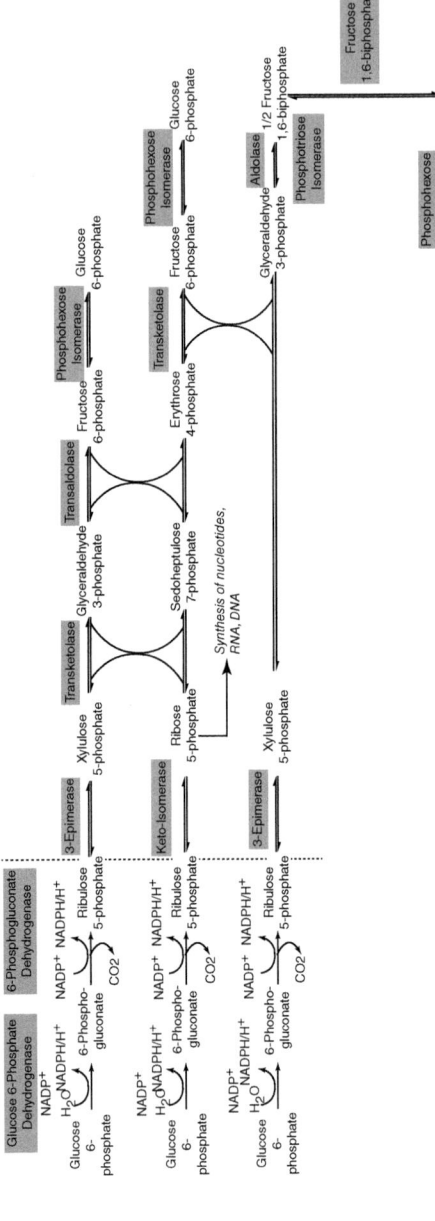

Fig. 1.19 The hexose monophosphate shunt (pentose phosphate pathway)

The non-oxidative phase occurs in all tissues, because all tissues have a need for ribose production.

Because glucose-6-phosphate is both a substrate and a product of this shunt, cells that do not carry out the oxidative phase simply proceed from the bottom to reach important intermediate substrates.

Glucose-6-phosphate dehydrogenase (G6PD) deficiency is the leading cause of hemolytic anemia and affects 100 million individuals worldwide. Without G6PD, erythrocytes are unable to generate NADPH, which is essential to reduce glutathione and thus prevent oxidative damage.

Insulin and Glucagon: Regulation of Glucose Metabolism

Insulin synthesis occurs in the pancreatic β-cells. Insulin is a peptide that is initially translated as preproinsulin. Preproinsulin is successively transformed to proinsulin by the formation of disulfide bonds and then to insulin and C-peptide by enzymatic cleavage:

$$\text{Preproinsulin} \rightarrow \text{Proinsulin} \rightarrow \text{Insulin} + \text{C}-\text{peptide}$$

Insulin secretion Glucose is taken up into a β-cell via a GLUT2 (insulin independent) transporter and metabolized, leading to ATP synthesis. Increased ATP levels lead to K$^+$ channels (Kir6.2) closing, leading to depolarization of the β-cell. Kir6.2 is associated with SUR1, the target of the class of antidiabetic drugs known as sulfonylureas. This leads to extracellular calcium influx and mobilization of intracellular calcium stores which leads to fusion of granules containing insulin with the plasma membrane. Thus insulin is released into the circulation.

Insulin action in muscle or fat Insulin binds to the insulin receptor, a receptor tyrosine kinase, leading to ATP dependent phosphorylation of the receptor itself (autophosphorylation). This activates the receptor, which then phosphorylates the IRSs (insulin receptor substrates). These lead to PI3 kinase activation and a number of signaling cascades. All of this leads to vesicles containing GLUT4 fusing with the plasma membrane, allowing glucose uptake into the cells.

Insulin action in the liver Insulin binds to the insulin receptor, leading to PI3K signaling as in muscle and fat. This leads to activation of phosphatases that downregulate the activity of glycogen phosphorylase and upregulate the activity of glycogen synthase. Similarly, gluconeogenesis is downregulated.

Diseases

Type 1 Diabetes Mellitus Autoimmune destruction of β-cells, requires insulin, prone to DKA, associated with MHC II genes.

Type 2 Diabetes Mellitus Insulin resistance, DKA unusual, polygenic.

Maturity Onset Diabetes of the Young (MODY) Caused by mutations in enzymes necessary for insulin secretion in the pancreas; displays a type 2 diabetes like phenotype.

The Metabolic Syndrome Insulin resistance, abdominal obesity, high TG + low HDL + high LDL, HTN, prothrombotic and proinflammatory.
  Obesity leads to type 2 diabetes via

1. Increased insulin resistance through hormonal signals released by abdominal fat, including resistin. Additionally, adiponectin is downregulated.
2. Inflammation: high CRP and IL-6 are correlated with developing diabetes, and mRNA analysis of fat from mice fed with a fatty diet showed increased NFkB levels. Simply activating NFkB in fat cells in mice (equivalent to fatty diet levels) leads to insulin resistance.

Fructose Metabolism

Fructose enters cells through GLUT5, after which it is phosphorylated by **fructokinase** to fructose-1-phoshphate. Fructose-1-phosphate is a direct substrate for **aldolase**, which cleaves to DHAP and glyceraldehyde. Glyceraldehyde is then converted to GAP by triose kinase (triokinase), and then GAP proceeds through the rest of glycolysis to produce pyruvate. Hence, fructose bypasses the key rate determining step of glycolysis, phosphofructokinase-1. Hence, fructose metabolism is much faster than glucose metabolism, leading to increased fatty acid synthesis and VLDL production in the liver, a possible cause of dyslipidemias. A summary of fructose metabolism is given in Fig. 1.20.

Important disorders in fructose metabolism:

- Essential fructosuria
  - Defect in fructokinase.
  - Benign and asymptomatic, although excess fructose accumulates in urine and blood.
- Fructose intolerance
  - Deficiency in aldolase B (recessive).
  - Accumulation of fructose-1-phosphate leads to decrease in available phosphate and subsequent inhibition of gluconeogenesis and glycogenolysis.
  - Symptoms include: hypoglycemia, jaundice, cirrhosis, hyperuricemia, can lead to hepatic failure and death.
  - Treatment: Avoid fructose and sucrose in diet.

1 Carbohydrate Metabolism

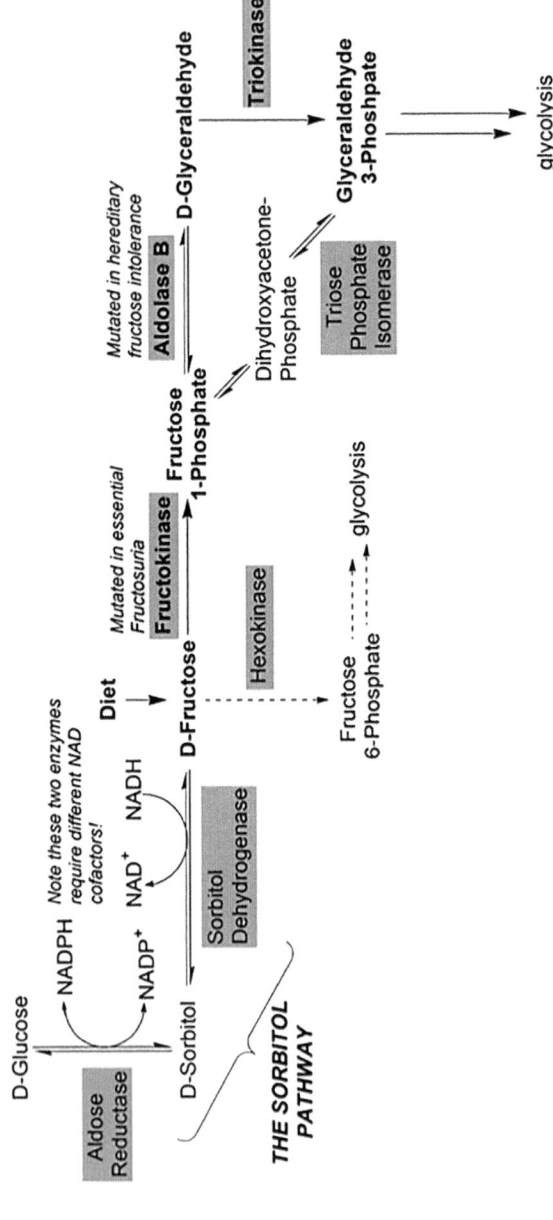

Fig. 1.20 Fructose metabolism

The Sorbitol Pathway

Both glucose and fructose can be converted to sorbitol through reduction. In glucose, the aldehyde at carbon 1 is reduced, while in fructose, the ketone at carbon 2 is reduced. These reactions are carried out by different enzymes. When glucose or fructose accumulates in cells, they can be shunted to sorbitol. The plasma membrane is impermeable to sorbitol, so sorbitol accumulates in the cell. If a sufficient quantity of sorbitol accumulates in the cell, leading to water influx and osmotic damage. ***Hyperglycemia as can occur in uncontrolled diabetes and fructose metabolism disorders are important causes of sorbitol accumulation, which can cause cataracts and erythrocyte damage. This is the major mechanism of cataract formation in diabetes.***

Galactose Metabolism

Galactose enters cells largely through the glucose transporters. It is phosphorylated to galactose-1-phosphate by **galactokinase**. It is then converted to UDP-galactose by **galactose-1-phosphate uridyltransferase**. UDP-glucose is then epimerized to UDP-glucose by **uridine diphosphogalactose-4 epimerase**. UDP-glucose can be used for glycogen synthesis as discussed earlier.

Important disorders of galactose metabolism:

1. Galactosemia results from galactose-1-phosphate uridyltransferase deficiency, resulting in galactosemia, galactosuria, jaundice, and diarrhea. The accumulation of toxic byproducts, including galactitol and galactose-1-phosphate, causes liver damage, cataracts, and mental retardation. The only treatment is to avoid dietary galactose and lactose.
2. Galactokinase deficiency results in a similar disease to galactosemia, causing galactosuria and galactosemia, with galactitol accumulation leading to similar effects.

Summary of Important disorders of galactose metabolism:

- Galactosemia
  - Deficiency in galactose-1-phosphate uridyltransferase (recessive).
  - Causes galactosemia and galactosuria, jaundice, diarrhea.
  - Accumulation of toxic substances, including galactitol and galactose-1-phosphate, causes liver damage, cataracts, and mental retardation.
  - Treatment: Avoid galactose and lactose in diet.
- Galactokinase deficiency—similar to Galactosemia
  - Causes galactosuria and galactosemia.
  - Galactitol accumulates, leading to cataract formation.

Biochemical Changes During Exercise

Exercise decreases blood insulin and increases blood glucagon, thus increasing glycogen phosphorylase activity and decreasing glycogen synthase activity. Exercise increases glucose transport in skeletal muscle by increasing surface GLUT4 levels through mechanisms independent of insulin signaling, possibly by activating adenosine monophosphate dependent kinase (AMPK), which then leads to phosphorylation of GLUT4 and membrane translocation. **Metformin, a major drug for type 2 diabetes, may act by inducing AMPK in muscle and liver. This is important, because in type 2 diabetes, insulin resistance leads to decreased rates of insulin mediated glucose uptake in skeletal muscle, so metformin may bypass insulin signaling to induce glucose uptake.**

- Effects of insulin and exercise.
  - Exercise decreases blood insulin, increases blood glucagon, increases glycogen. Phosphorylase and glycogen synthase activity (glycogen breakdown for fuel and synthesis for replenishment take place at the same time).
  - Insulin also stimulates glycogen synthase (via PI3K and PP1G).

- Exercise and insulin increase glucose transport in skeletal muscle by increasing surface GLUT4 levels (and thus decrease blood glucose).
  - They do so via different mechanisms (they are additive and exercise-stimulated changes in glucose transport can happen in the absence of insulin)!
  - This is important, because in type 2 diabetes, insulin resistance leads to decreased rates of insulin mediated glucose uptake in skeletal muscle.
  - Insulin acts via the insulin receptor, IRSs, PI3K, and perhaps Akt and PKCs.
  - One of the mechanisms whereby exercise increases GLUT4 levels at the cell surface is increased AMPK activity.
    AMPK.
      "Fuel sensor"—metabolite sensing protein (activated by AMP).
      Activated by phosphorylation by AMPKK and also directly by AMP; AMP also activates AMPKK.
      Leads to increased glucose transport by increasing GLUT4 translocation to the plasma membrane.

Metformin, a major drug for type 2 diabetes, may act by inducing AMPK in muscle and liver.

Important Diseases of Carbohydrate Metabolism

Major Metabolic Diseases

Type 1 Diabetes mellitus involves the autoimmune destruction of β-cells. Patients require insulin and are prone to diabetic ketoacidosis (DKA). There is a genetic associated with MHC II genes.

Type 2 Diabetes mellitus results from insulin resistance. DKA is unusual, although patients can suffer from the hyperosmolar hyperglycemic state (HHS). It is polygenic in inheritance pattern.

Maturity onset diabetes of the young (MODY) is caused by mutations in enzymes necessary for insulin secretion in the pancreas and displays a type 2 diabetes like phenotype.

The metabolic syndrome consists of insulin resistance, abdominal obesity, dyslipidemia (high triglycerides, low HDL, high LDL), hypertension, and a prothrombotic and proinflammatory state.

Obesity leads to type 2 diabetes via

1. increased insulin resistance through hormonal signals released by abdominal fat, including resistin. Additionally, adiponectin, a protective hormone, is downregulated.
2. inflammation as a part of the metabolic syndrome: high CRP and IL-6 are correlated with developing diabetes.

Some Important Enzyme Deficiencies in Carbohydrate Metabolism

Aldolase A Deficiency—results in hemolytic anemia

Pyruvate Dehydrogenase Deficiency—results in congenital lactic acidosis

Glycogen Storage Diseases

Glucose-6-Phosphate Dehydrogenase Deficiency—the leading cause of hemolytic anemia

Essential Fructosuria (Fructokinase Deficiency)—results in benign fructosuria

Aldolase B Deficiency (Fructose Intolerance)—results in cirrhosis, jaundice, and liver failure

Galactosemia (Galactose-1-phosphate Uridyltransferase Deficiency)—results in galactitol accumulation, with liver damage, mental retardation, and cataracts

Galactokinase Deficiency—results in similar symptoms to galactosemia.

Lipid Metabolism

2

Biologically Important Lipids

Fatty Acids Hydrocarbon chains with a terminal carboxyl group.

Saturated Fatty Acids Fatty acids that contain no double bonds (all single bonds). Saturated fatty acids tend to have relatively high melting points and are generally solid at room temperature. *The most common saturated fatty acid is* ***palmitic acid****, which contains 16 carbons, shown in* Fig. 2.1.

Monounsaturated Fatty Acids Fatty acids that contain a single double bond (**generally cis**).

Polyunsaturated Fatty Acids Fatty acids that contain multiple double bonds (**generally cis**).

There are multiple classification systems for unsaturated fatty acids, and you should be familiar with them because they occur repeatedly in various sources. The simplest, and most common, is

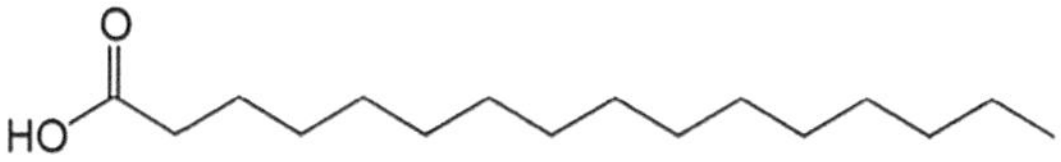

Fig. 2.1 Palmitic acid

V. Yanamadala, *Essential Medical Biochemistry and Metabolic Disease*, https://doi.org/10.1007/978-3-031-59394-9_2

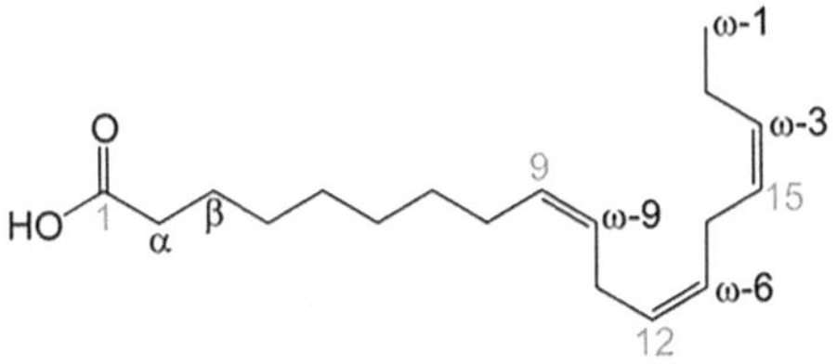

Fig. 2.2 α-linolenic acid

the ω system. The *ω-carbon of a fatty acid is the terminal carbon. This is also known as ω-1. The carbons are then numbered toward the carboxy-terminus as ω-2, ω-3, ω-4, etc. as shown below in the red numbering scheme. The fatty acids are classified based on the first carbon at which a double bond occurs. For example, all ω-3 fatty acids have a double bond between the ω-3 and ω-4 carbons. α-linolenic acid, an example of an ω-3 fatty acid, is shown in Fig. 2.2.*

The other classification system relies on specifying the length of the carbon chain, the number of double bonds, and the carbons at which the double bonds occur. This system counts the carbon of the carboxyl group as carbon 1 and then counts toward the end of the chain (blue numbering system above). For example, α-linolenic acid above would be named 18:3;9,12,15 because it has 18 carbons, 3 double bonds, and the double bonds occur at carbon 9, 12, and 15 of the blue numbering system. Both numbering systems exist and you should be familiar with them, although you do not have to memorize the specific nomenclatures for particular fatty acids. It is, however, worthwhile to familiarize yourselves with a number of important ω-3, ω-6, and ω-9 fatty acids that are of biological importance.

Essential Fatty Acids

There are three fatty acids that are considered essential fatty acids because the human body cannot synthesize them. These are **linoleic acid**, **α-linolenic acid**, and **arachidonic acid**. Arachidonic acid is technically not an essential fatty acid because the body can synthesize it from linolenic acid; however, deficiencies can occur, and arachidonic acid becomes essential when dietary intake of linoleic acid is insufficient.

Harmful Fats

Trans Fatty Acid: An unsaturated fatty acid that contains one or more trans double bond. These are rare in nature and are usually the product of **partial hydrogenation**, an industrial process that serves to solidify liquid fats.

Simple Fatty Acids and Nutrition

Monounsaturated and polyunsaturated fatty acids appear to have a number of health benefits. These include lowering the risk of atherosclerosis and coronary heart disease.

Saturated fatty acids and trans fatty acids appear to have a number of detrimental effects. These include increased risk of atherosclerosis and coronary heart disease (by increasing plasma LDL levels, reducing plasma HDL levels (only trans fats), and overall increasing the LDL/HDL ratio).

Eicosapentaenoic acid (EPA) are ω-3 fatty acids present in fish oils that have been promoted recently as having anti-inflammatory effects. This will be described subsequently in the discussion of eicosanoids.

Docosahexaenoic acid (DHA) are another class of ω-3 fatty acids present in fish oils that have been promoted recently as necessary for proper brain and retina function. There is evidence that patients with *retinitis pigmentosa* are deficient in DHA.

Simple Lipids   Esters of fatty acids with various alcohols.

Fats/Oils: Esters of fatty acids with glycerol.
    Monoacylglycerols (monoglycerides)
    Diacylglycerols (diglycerides)
    Triacylglycerols (triglycerides)

Fig. 2.3 A simple fat

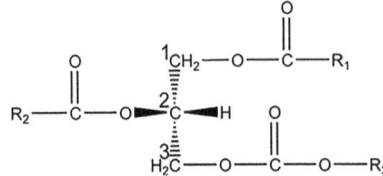

Waxes: Esters of fatty acid with high weight monohydric alcohols.

Interesterified fat.

The glycerol backbone has a nomenclature system in which the carbons are labeled sn1, sn2, and sn3 as shown in Fig. 2.3.

Because enzymes are chiral, they will usually act upon one of the three fatty acid chains of a triacylglycerol. This is especially important within the context of pancreatic lipases that digest lipids by selectively cleaving particular fatty acids from the glycerol backbone, a topic that is generally covered in more detail in gastrointestinal physiology courses.

Complex Lipids Modified esters of fatty acids.

Glycerophospholipids (phospholipids) consist of two fatty acids attached to a glycerol backbone at the sn1 and sn2 positions and a phosphate molecule attached at the sn3 position. The glycerophospholipid is named according to the group (R) attached to the phosphate. A typical glycerophospholipid is shown in Fig. 2.4.

Phosphatidic Acid (Phosphatidate)—R = H

Phosphatidylcholines (lecithins)—R = choline $CH_2CH_2N(CH_3)_3^+$.

Dipalmitoyl lecithin: A phosphatidylcholine with two palmitic acid side chains; this is pulmonary surfactant, the absence of which results in ***Adult Respiratory Distress Syndrome (ARDS).***

Phosphatidylethanolamines—R = ethanolamine $CH_2CH_2NH_3^+$.

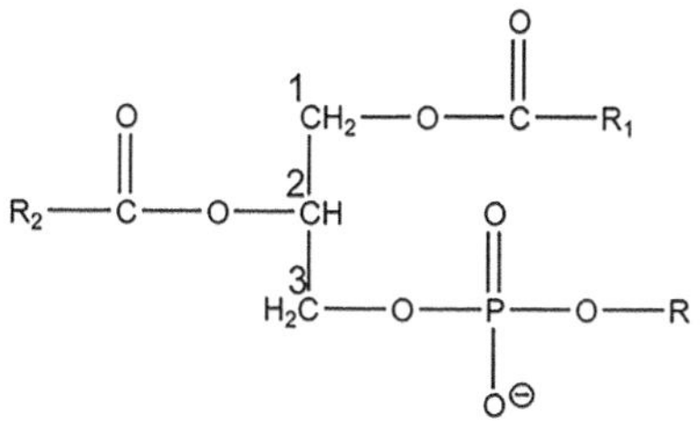

Simple Fatty Acids and Nutrition

Fig. 2.4 The general phospholipid

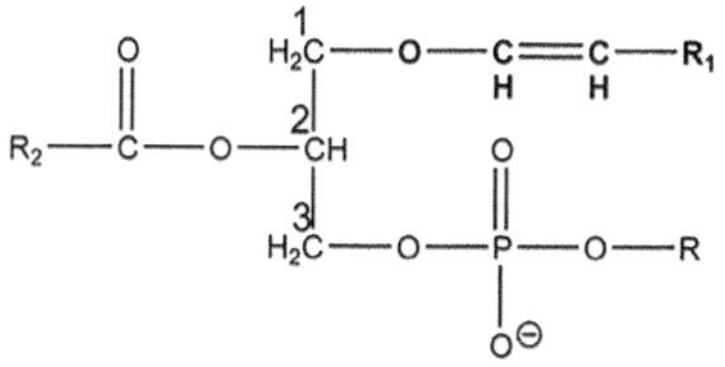

Fig. 2.5 The plasmalogen

Phosphatidylserines—R = serine
Phosphatidylinositols—R = myoinositol
Cardiolipins: A diphosphatidylglycerol; these are the major lipids of mitochondrial membranes.

Plasmalogens: A modified glycerophospholipid-like molecule that has a **fatty ether** linkage at the sn1 position of the glycerol. This is shown in Fig. 2.5 in bold. Plasmalogens constitute as much as 10% of the phospholipids of the brain and muscle. Plasmalogens may also contain choline, ethanolamine, serine, or inositol, as the R group on the phosphate and are named accordingly.

Phosphatidalethanolamine: Largely found in the brain and nervous tissues

Phosphatidalcholine: Largely found in the heart

Multiple sclerosis is a demyelinating disorder of the brain, the symptoms of which result from the loss of phospholipids and <u>ethanolamine plasmalogen</u> (phosphatidalethanolamine) from the myelin of the white matter of the brain.

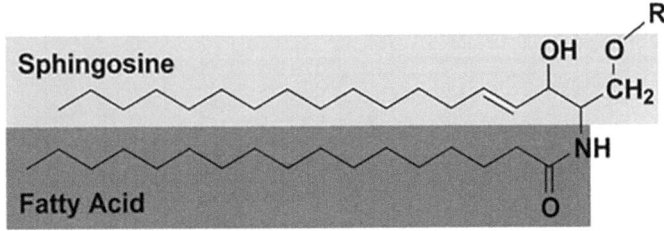

Fig. 2.6 The sphingolipid

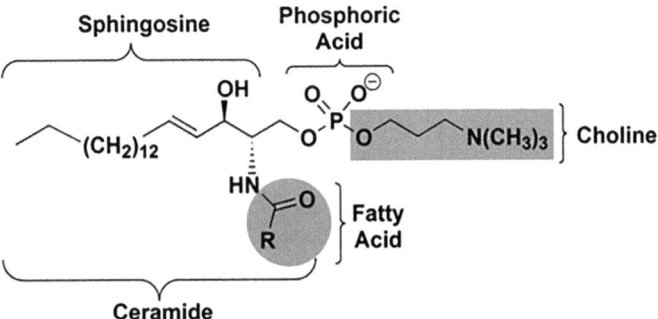

Fig. 2.7 The sphingomyelin

Sphingolipids Esters of fatty acids that contain a molecule of sphingosine in place of the glycerol backbone of fats and glycerophospholipids. To the sphingosine backbone is attached one fatty acid and one variable group (**R**). The sphingosine backbone and fatty acid together are referred to as **ceramide**. The general structure of sphingolipids is shown in Fig. 2.6.

Sphingomyelins—R = phosphorylcholine; these are present in the myelin sheaths of neurons and a structure is shown in Fig. 2.7.

Glycolipids (Glycosphingolipids): *All* glycolipids have a ceramide backbone and are hence more properly classified as glycosphingolipids. These are sphingolipids in which the R group is a monosaccharide or oligosaccharide.

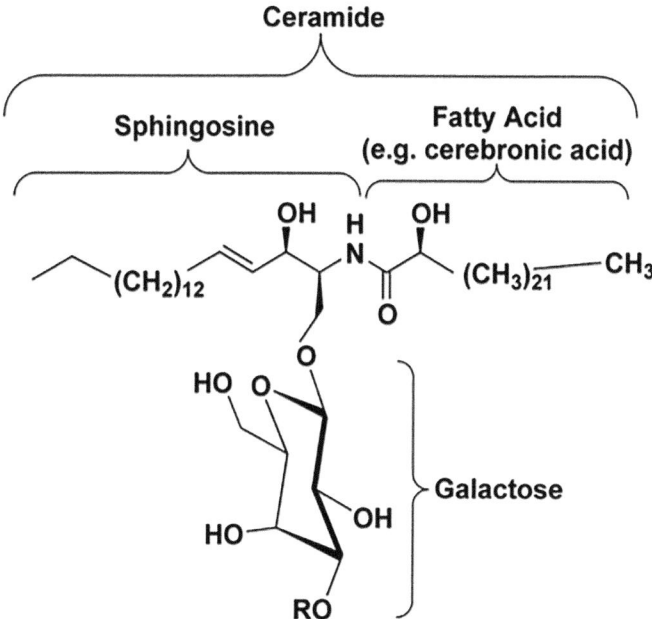

Fig. 2.8 The glycolipid

Galactosylceramide—R = galactose; found in abundance in the brain and other nervous tissues and shown in Fig. 2.8.

Gangliosides—R = oligosaccharide that contains a sialic acid (such as neuraminidic acid—NeuAc). Gangliosides are found in neurons in high concentrations and are also found in various other tissues, where they serve as cell surface recognition molecules and as cell surface receptors. The G_{M1} ganglioside is shown in Fig. 2.9.

Sulfosphingolipids.
Aminosphingolipids.

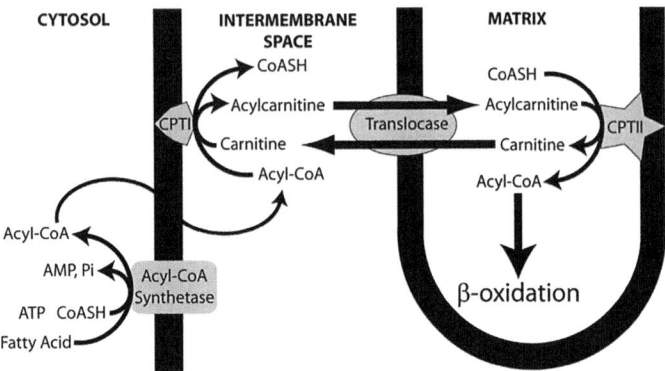

Fig. 2.9 The carnitine shuttle allows for the transport of activated fatty acids in the form of acyl-CoA into the mitochondrial matrix, where oxidation occurs. CPTI is carnitine palmitoyl transferase I and is the rate limiting step of the shuttle. CPTII is carnitine palmitoyl transferase II

Oxidation of Fatty Acids

Transport into the Mitochondrion: The Carnitine Shuttle

Long chain fatty acids are activated by CoA in the cytosol by **acyl-coA synthetase**, an enzyme of the outer mitochondrial membrane, in an ATP dependent fashion. *This is the one step in fatty acid degradation that expends ATP*. This step requires the equivalent of **two ATPs**. This is because ATP is converted to AMP and pyrophosphate during this process, with pyrophosphate further degraded by pyrophosphatase into two inorganic phosphates. I do not discuss the details of this process here.

Acyl-CoA are freely permeable through the outer mitochondrial membrane. However, they cannot penetrate the inner mitochondrial membrane. This is the role of the **carnitine shuttle**, shown in Fig. 2.10. Carnitine acts as a shuttle protein that transfers the fatty acid across the inner mitochondrial membrane. Carnitine palmitoyltransferase I serves to exchange an acyl group to form an acylcarnitine from the acyl-CoA within the intermem-

Oxidation of Fatty Acids

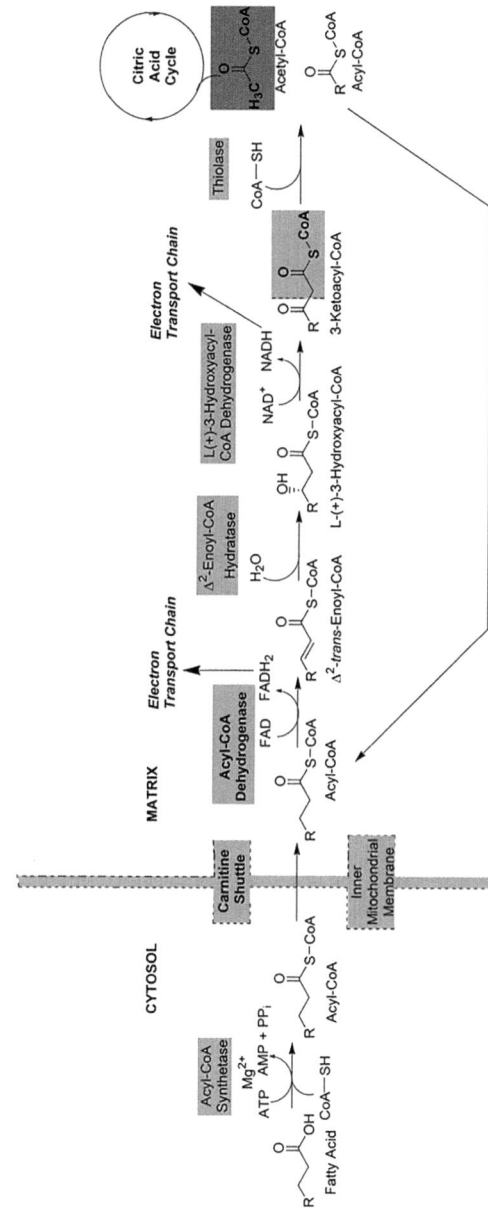

Fig. 2.10 β-oxidation of fatty acids

brane space. **Carnitine Acylcarnitine Translocase** then allows the acylcarnitine to enter the mitochondrial matrix in exchange for a free carnitine molecule. Within the matrix, **carnitine palmitoyltransferase II** then serves to convert acylcarnitine back to acyl-CoA. The acyl-CoA is then metabolized within the mitochondrial matrix by a process known as β-oxidation.

Short and medium chain fatty acids (less than 12 carbons) freely penetrate through the inner mitochondrial membrane in their nonionized forms and are simply activated by an **acyltransferase** to the acyl-CoA within the mitochondrial matrix.

Carnitine Palmitoyltransferase I is generally regarded as the rate-limiting enzyme of fatty acid oxidation. As such, it is highly regulated. Malonyl-CoA, a key intermediate in fatty acid synthesis, inhibits CPTI, thus inhibiting oxidation of fatty acids, while synthesis is actively taking place. Insulin also influences the activity of CPTI, as described subsequently.

Carnitine deficiencies can result in a syndrome called fasting hypoketotic hypoglycemia. The syndrome is associated with muscle weakness and myoglobinuria after prolonged exercise (as muscle breaks down, releasing myoglobin). The same symptoms are seen with genetic defects in the carnitine palmitoyltransferase I.

β-Oxidation

Within the mitochondrial matrix, fatty acids are oxidized to two carbons at a time from the carboxyl end to form units of acetyl-CoA. This acetyl-CoA then enters the TCA cycle. The bond between the α and the β carbons is cleaved, hence the name β-oxidation. The general scheme of β-oxidation is shown in Fig. 2.11.

Congenital defects in the **medium chain acyl-CoA dehydrogenase (MCAD)** lead to the accumulation of medium chain fatty acids in the mitochondria. Because medium chain fatty acids are an important source of acetyl-CoA for gluconeogenesis, this disorder is also associated with *fasting hypoketotic hypoglycemia*.

Oxidation of Fatty Acids

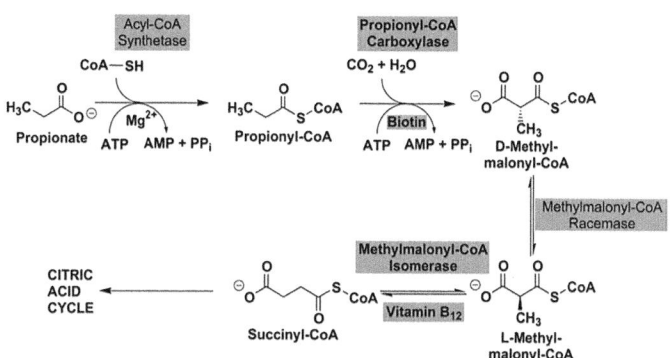

Fig. 2.11 Propionic acid is metabolized to succinyl-CoA, an intermediate of the citric acid cycle, by a series of enzymes that require biotin and vitamin B12 as cofactors

Symptoms can include vomiting, coma, and death due to insufficient energy delivery to the brain.

As you might imagine, the oxidation of an even chain fatty acid of n carbons yields a $n/2$ acetyl-CoA molecules. The oxidation of an odd chain fatty acid of n carbons results in the formation of $(n - 3)/2$ acetyl-CoA molecules plus one molecule of propionyl-CoA. molecules plus one molecule of propionyl-CoA. This is because the final three-carbon chain cannot be further metabolized.

Even chain fatty acid (n carbons): $n/2$ acetyl Co-A

Odd chain fatty acid (n carbons): $(n - 3)/2$ acetyl Co-A + propionyl-CoA

The metabolism of propionyl-CoA is shown in Fig. 2.12. This is a pathway with several key points to remember. This pathway is one of the two pathways in human metabolism that requires vitamin B12 (the other is the conversion of the amino acid methionine to the amino acid cysteine, which we will cover in Chap. 3). Propionyl-CoA is converted to D-methylmalonyl-CoA by **Propionyl-CoA Carboxylase**, an enzyme that requires **biotin** as a cofactor. D-Methylmalonyl-CoA is converted to its enantiomer, L-methylmalonyl-CoA, by methylmalonyl-CoA racemase. Then L-methylmalonyl-CoA is converted to succinyl-CoA by

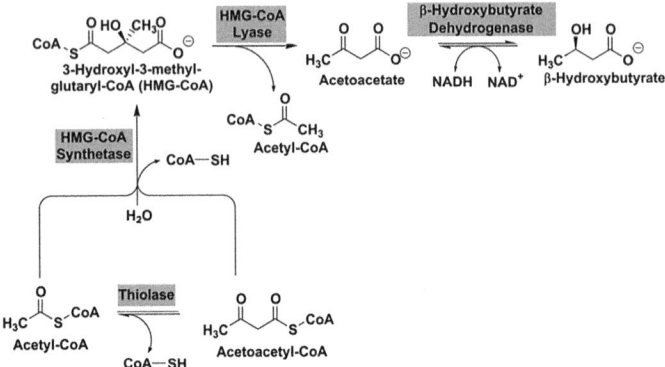

Fig. 2.12 Ketone bodies are generated from acetyl-CoA in the liver as alternative sources of energy when glucose stores are low

Methylmalonyl-CoA Isomerase, the enzyme which requires vitamin B12. Succinyl-CoA then enters the TCA.

Because propionate can yield succinyl-CoA, it is eventually metabolized to oxaloacetate in the TCA. Because oxaloacetate is an intermediate in gluconeogenesis, propionate can be converted to glucose! This is the only means by which fatty acid oxidation can be glucogenic. Otherwise, acetyl-CoA produced by all other fatty acid synthesis cannot form glucose and can only be converted into ketone bodies.

Inactivating mutations in **propionyl-CoA carboxylase** result in **propionic acidemia**, while mutations in **methylmalonyl-CoA isomerase (methylmalonyl-CoA mutase)** result in **methylmalonic acidemia**. Both of these conditions are associated with hyperammonemia, which can lead to **encephalopathy** and **severe mental disorders** (see Laura's lectures on amino acid metabolism for more on hyperammonemia).

Energy Accounting

Each two carbon fragment of an **even chain fatty acid** yields one NADH and one $FADH_2$ in the process of being converted to acetyl-CoA. This is the equivalent of a net five ATP. Additionally, each acetyl-CoA produces 3 NADH, 1 FADH$_2$, and 1 ATP (or GTP) through the TCA, yielding an additional 12 ATP. *Hence, each 2 carbon fragment of a fatty acid yields 17 ATP.* Fatty acid metabolism requires activation at the beginning, which expends two ATPs. Hence:

Number of ATP Produced = $17^* (n/2) - 2$ n = number of carbons

Oxidation of Unsaturated Fatty Acids

Unsaturated fatty acids are metabolized just like saturated fatty acids until the first unsaturated carbon comes to the β-position. At this point, the cis double bond is isomerized to a trans double bond by **Δ^3-cis → Δ^2-trans-enoyl-CoA isomerase**. As you imagine, the resulting substrate now looks exactly like a substrate for **Δ^2-trans-enoyl-CoA hydratase** and continues through the normal β oxidation pathway for saturated fatty acids.

Peroxisomal Fatty Acid Metabolism

Very long chain fatty acids (greater than 20 carbons) cannot be oxidized directly in the mitochondrion. Very long chain fatty acids (VLCFAs) are oxidized first in peroxisomes to octanoyl-CoA (an eight carbon fatty acid), which can then be metabolized in the mitochondrion. VLCFAs enter the peroxisome through a transporter known as **ALDP**. Once inside the peroxisome, VLCFAs are metabolized by β-oxidation by an FAD dependent enzyme called **acyl-coA oxidase** that leads to the formation of acetyl-CoA and H$_2$O$_2$. *Notice the distinction here between mitochondrial fatty acid oxidation that requires FAD and NAD+ vs. peroxisomal fatty acid oxidation, which only requires FAD.* Octanoyl-CoA then exits the peroxisome through ALDP.

Inactivating mutations in ALDP lead to a disorder known as X-linked adrenoleukodystrophy, in which VLCFAs accumulate

in various tissues, leading to progressive brain damage, adrenal gland dysfunction, and eventually death.

Inactivating mutations in genes involved in the formation of peroxisomes, known as peroxins (PEX1, PEX2, PEX3, PEX5, PEX6, and others), result in <u>Zellweger Syndrome (cerebrohepatorenal syndrome)</u>, which is characterized by liver failure, mental retardation, and seizures.

Ketone Body Formation

While fatty acid oxidation yields large quantities of ATP that can be used for gluconeogenesis in the liver, another important metabolic end product of fatty acid oxidation are ketone bodies. Because gluconeogenic substrates, such as amino acids, are depleted over time, ketone bodies yield another energy source that can be shuttled into the bloodstream by the liver for use by other tissues, including the brain. The major utilizable ketone bodies are **acetoacetate** and **β-hydroxybutyrate (3-hydroxybutyrate)**. Additionally, acetoacetate may spontaneously decompose to **acetone**, releasing carbon dioxide. Acetoacetate can be converted to acetyl-CoA for use in the respiratory chain. β-hydroxybutyrate is first converted to acetoacetate and then metabolized to acetyl-CoA. Hence, these provide important alternative energy sources in the absence of glucose.

As the serum fatty acid concentration increases, the fatty acid metabolism in the liver exceeds the capacity of the TCA and electron transport chain. Thus, acetyl-CoA is diverted into ketone body formation by the pathway shown in Fig. 2.13. **HMG-CoA Synthase** is the rate-limiting enzyme in the process of ketone body formation.

The balance between acetoacetate and β-hydroxybutyrate is determined by the $NADH:NAD^+$ ratio within the tissues, especially the liver. High NADH levels result in the formation of β-hydroxybutyrate, while low NADH levels result primarily in the formation of acetoacetate. Both are utilizable by extrahepatic tissues. Acetoacetate and β-hydroxybutyrate are interconverted

Oxidation of Fatty Acids

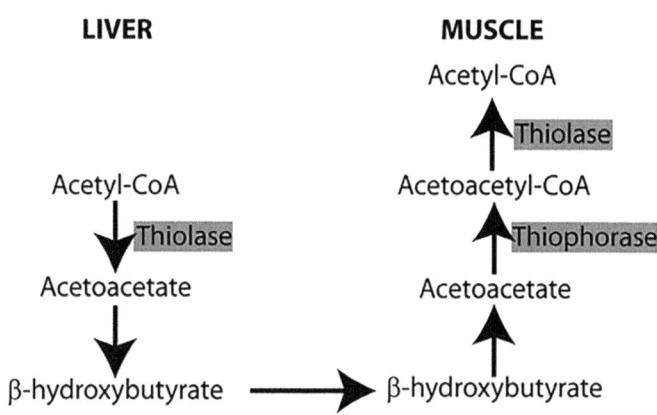

Fig. 2.13 Ketone body cycling

within the mitochondrial matrix by **β-hydroxybutyrate dehydrogenase (3-hydroxybutyrate dehydrogenase).**

The liver releases ketone bodies (acetoacetate and β-hydroxybutyrate) into the circulation. Extrahepatic tissues possess **CoA Transferase (thiophorase)**, which converts **acetoacetate** to **acetoacetyl-CoA**, which can then transformed to acetyl-CoA by thiolase and used to generate NADH and $FADH_2$ in the TCA. This process is shown in Fig. 2.14. The liver does not possess thiophorase and thus cannot metabolize ketone bodies because it cannot make the activated acetoacetyl-CoA from acetoacetate. The acetoacetyl-CoA generated in the liver to produce ketone bodies is made by thiolase from acetyl-CoA, which is primarily generated from fatty acid oxidation.

Diabetic Ketoacidosis is a condition associated with <u>hyperglycemia</u>. In this case, the absolute lack of insulin results in increased lipolysis and release of fatty acids from adipose tissue and increased fatty oxidation in the liver. This uncontrolled fatty acid metabolism leads to the accumulation of ketone bodies in the blood. Because these are acids, an acidosis develops that can be fatal if not treated immediately by insulin administration. Thus, ketone body production normally occurs in hypoglycemic states as a means to provide other sources of fuel to the body's

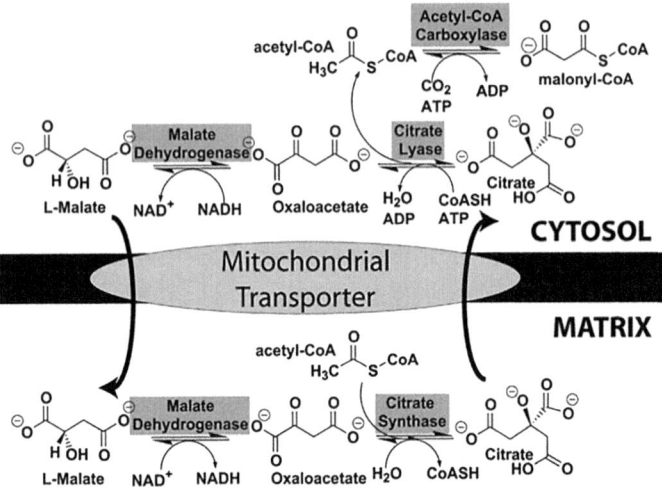

Fig. 2.14 The citrate shuttle mediates transport of acetyl-CoA from the mitochondrial matrix to the cytosol for fatty acid synthesis

tissues. Here in DKA, ketone bodies are pathologically produced in the setting of elevated glucose levels because of the absence of insulin mediated suppression of fatty acid metabolism.

Ketoacidosis can be diagnosed by examining urine ketone levels. Acetone and Acetoacetate are detected by urine dipstick. However, β-hydroxybutyrate is not detected by urine dipstick! This is important because, as you administer insulin, the patient begins to recover and fewer ketone bodies are produced. This means that less fatty acid oxidation is occurring and thus less NADH accumulates in the liver. This leads to the reoxidation of remaining β-hydroxybutyrate back to acetoacetate. Thus, in the early stages of recovery, blood and urine β-hydroxybutyrate levels drop and acetoacetate levels rise. *Thus, the patient may paradoxically appear to be doing worse if you look at urine dipstick to monitor progress! Therefore, a measure of blood ketones is often conducted simultaneously.*

Lipogenesis (Fatty Acid Synthesis)

While fatty acid oxidation occurs within the mitochondrial matrix, fatty acid synthesis (lipogenesis) occurs within the cytosol. This physical separation of fatty acid oxidation and synthesis allows for the independent control of both processes according to the needs of the tissue. **Acetyl-CoA** serves as the starting material and **palmitic acid** is the end point of cytosolic fatty acid synthesis.

Remember that acetyl-CoA generated by pyruvate dehydrogenase is trapped within the mitochondrial matrix and is not permeable across the inner mitochondrial membrane. Hence, another shuttle, the **citrate shuttle**, is necessary to transfer acetyl-CoA equivalents across the inner mitochondrial membrane. Here, acetyl-CoA and oxaloacetate are transformed into citrate by citrate synthase, and citrate diffuses into the cytosol. **Citrate lyase** then catalyzes the formation of acetyl-CoA and oxaloacetate in the cytosol, expending a molecule of ATP. This acetyl-CoA is then used for fatty acid synthesis, first being transformed into **malonyl-CoA** by **acetyl-CoA carboxylase** in an ATP dependent manner, before being polymerized by **fatty acid synthase**. *Acetyl-CoA Carboxylase is the rate-limiting step of fatty acid synthesis and is thus the most regulated step of the process.* A general schematic of fatty acid synthesis is shown in Fig. 2.15.

In the presence of insulin, acetyl-CoA carboxylase is dephosphorylated and thus activated, leading to increased fatty acid synthesis. Glucagon inhibits fatty acid synthesis by causing the phosphorylation of acetyl-CoA carboxylase.

Fatty acid synthase is a multienzyme complex that transforms 2 carbon building blocks into the 16 carbon saturated fatty acid palmitate. Fatty acid synthesis is in many ways an imperfect mirror image of β-oxidation. While the enzymes that catalyze the two pathways are completely different, the biochemical reactions are very similar—the long chain of palmitate is built up in units of two carbons just as fatty acids are oxidized by breaking off units of two carbons. Of note, the first two carbons in palmitate are derived from a molecule of acetyl-CoA, while all subsequent two

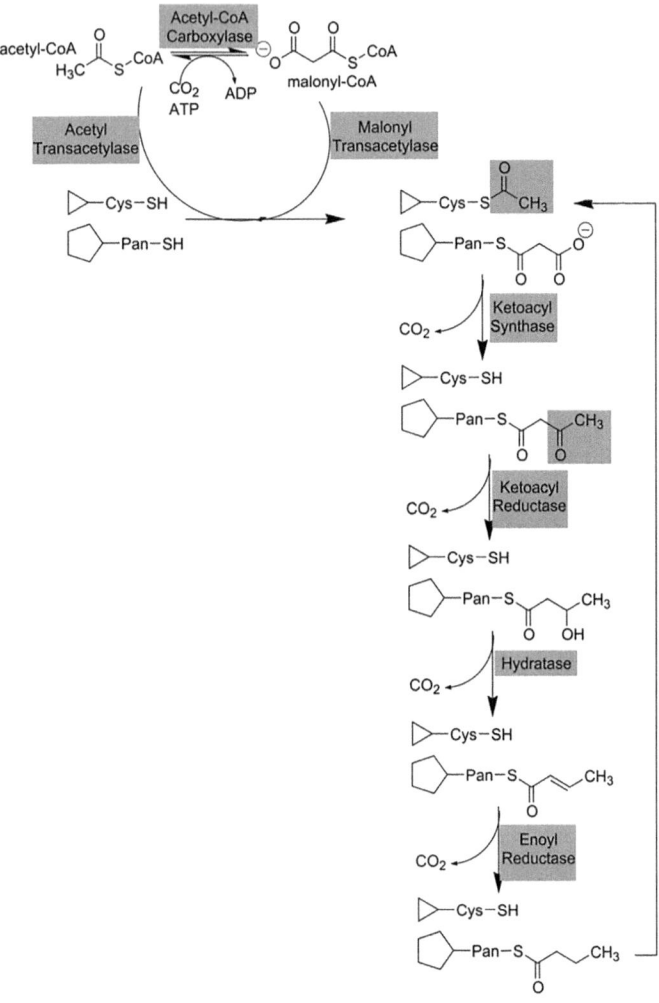

Fig. 2.15 Fatty acid synthesis

carbon fragments come from malonyl-CoA, with decarboxylation of malonyl-CoA yielding the energetic driving force that propels fatty acid synthesis. The first two carbons of the fatty acid chain come from a molecule of acetyl-CoA.

Of important note, while β-oxidation produces NADH from NAD^+, fatty acid synthesis uses NADPH and yields $NADP^+$. One of the major uses of NADPH, as discussed in the carbohydrate metabolism review sheet, is fatty acid synthesis. Without a functional pentose phosphate pathway (HMP Shunt), fatty acid synthesis is impaired. Fatty acid synthesis primarily occurs in the liver, while fat storage primarily occurs in adipose tissue. As we will learn in the section on lipid transport, the primary function of VLDL is the transport of lipids produced in the liver to the rest of the body.

I present the pathway of fatty acid synthesis in Fig. 2.15, not because you are expected to memorize the steps of this pathway, but because it is worthwhile to familiarize yourselves with the process. *What you should know, however, is that the principal product of <u>cytosolic</u> fatty acid synthesis is <u>palmitic acid</u> (the 16 carbon saturated fatty acid).* Notice here once again that this is a cyclical process, just like β-oxidation. The whole process is catalyzed by a single multi-domain enzyme, **fatty acid synthase**.

Fatty Acid Elongation

The body has a need to produce fatty acids that are longer than 16 carbons, of course. Additionally, it has a need to elongate preexisting fatty acids. Elongation is one important pathway by which essential dietary fatty acids are transformed into other physiologically important fatty acids. This elongation takes place in the **endoplasmic reticulum**. The **microsomal fatty acid elongase system** elongates saturated and unsaturated fatty acids that are at least ten carbons long in two carbon segments using malonyl-CoA and NADPH in a manner similar to that used by fatty acid synthase. This system produces the very long chain fatty acids (C22 and C24) that are necessary for **myelin formation** and other processes.

Synthesis of Monounsaturated and Polyunsaturated Fatty Acids

The liver is capable of synthesizing several nonessential monounsaturated and polyunsaturated fatty acids. The liver uses **desaturases**, enzymes that utilize molecular O_2 and NADH to desaturate a preformed saturated fatty acid. These enzymes are also found within the endoplasmic reticulum **microsomal system**. Using the desaturase and elongase system in conjunction, the liver can synthesize a variety of monounsaturated and polyunsaturated fatty acids.

Regulation of Fatty Acid Synthesis

The majority of regulation occurs at the step of **acetyl-CoA Carboxylase**. Phosphorylation of this enzyme leads to its inactivation, while dephosphorylation leads to its activation. As expected, glucagon activates PKA and other kinases such as AMPK, which in turn phosphorylate and inactivate this enzyme. Conversely, insulin activates various protein phosphatases that dephosphorylate this enzyme and lead to its activation. Thus, insulin glucagon inhibits lipogenesis, while insulin promotes lipogenesis.

Insulin in Fatty Acid Metabolism

1. Insulin stimulates lipogenesis by
   (a) Increasing acetyl-CoA carboxylase activity by causing its dephosphorylation.
   (b) Increasing the transport of glucose into adipose tissue and thus increasing the availability of substrates for lipogenesis.
   (c) Increases pyruvate dehydrogenase activity in adipose tissue by increasing the activity of PDH phosphatase and thus increasing the levels of dephosphorylated active

PDH. This leads to the increased production of acetyl-CoA, the major substrate for lipogenesis.
2. Insulin inhibits fatty acid catabolism
   (a) By decreasing **hormone sensitive lipase** activity. HSL is an enzyme in adipose tissue that releases free fatty acids from triglycerides, allowing them to diffuse to the liver for metabolism.
   (b) By regulating in the liver the activity of **carnitine palmitoyltransferase I (CPTI)**, a key enzyme that allows fatty acids to enter the mitochondrion.
      - Indirectly by increasing fatty acid synthesis and thus the levels of **malonyl-CoA**, an important allosteric inhibitor of CPTI.
      - Directly through as yet poorly understood pathways.

Glucagon and Epinephrine largely have the opposite effects in all of the above pathways.

Comparing and Contrasting Fatty Acid Synthesis and Oxidation

Fatty acid synthesis and oxidation are compared and contrasted in Table 2.1, in which the key aspects of both processes are also summarized.

Table 2.1 Comparing and contrasting fatty acid synthesis and oxidation

	Fatty acid synthesis	Fatty acid oxidation
Purpose	Energy storage	Energy generation
Final product	Triacylglycerol (three fatty acids attached to glycerol)	Full oxidation: 9 kcal/g of fat or 131 ATP from 1 molecule of palmityl CoA (16 carbons)
		Ketone bodies: generated by the liver to be converted to ATP in other tissues
		Glycerol is reused to produce glucose through gluconeogenesis

(continued)

Table 2.1 (continued)

	Fatty acid synthesis	Fatty acid oxidation
Tissues involved	Liver (mostly), lactating mammary glands, adipose tissue	Liver, cardiomyocytes, myocytes, and other tissues
Subcellular localization	Cytosol	Mitochondria
Membrane transport	Citrate is transported across the mitochondrial membrane to the cytosol by the citrate shuttle	Long chain fatty acids are carried into the mitochondria by the carnitine shuttle
Cofactors	NADPH, ATP	NAD^+, FAD
Hormonal regulation	Stimulated by insulin	Inhibited by insulin
	Inhibited by glucagon	Stimulated by glucagon
Other regulation	Inhibited by epinephrine	

Metabolism of Glycerolipids

Once fatty acids are synthesized or absorbed in the intestine, they must be transformed into the various simple lipids. The acylglycerols (fats and oils) require three fatty acids and a glycerol backbone. The glycerol backbone is derived from glycerol-3-phosphate, which is formed from dihydroxyacetone phosphate (DHAP), a glycolysis intermediate, by **glycerol-3-phosphate dehydrogenase**. Fatty acids are activated by **acyl-CoA synthetase** to acyl-CoAs. Two acyl-CoAs can then combine with the glycerol-3-phosphate to form a **phosphatidate**. This process is shown in Fig. 2.16. Phosphatidic acid is the intermediate that leads to the synthesis of triacylglycerols (triglycerides), the ultimate storage form of fatty acids in adipose tissue. This is achieved by **phosphatidate phosphohydrolase** and **diacylglycerol acyltransferase**.

Phosphatidic acid also serves as the intermediate for the synthesis of the phospholipids (glycerophospholipids). Choline and ethanolamine are activated to **CDP-choline** and **CDP-ethanolamine** and these are conjugated to phosphatidic acid to

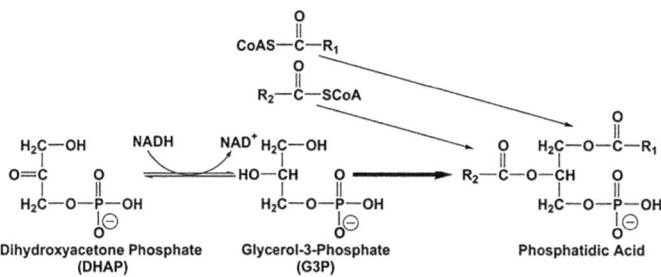

Fig. 2.16 Synthesis of phosphatidic acid, the backbone of glycerolipids

yield the respective phospholipids. This is a common theme that we have encountered before in glycogen synthesis—activation through nucleotidation. Phosphatidylserine is formed from phosphatidylethanolamine by a replacement reaction in which free serine replaces ethanolamine.

Phospholipids are degraded by **phospholipases**, which catalyze the hydrolysis of the fatty acid residue from the glycerol backbone. There are a number of phospholipases involved in cellular signaling cascades and others that are involved in digestion.

Metabolism of Sphingolipids

Ceramide is synthesized within the endoplasmic reticulum. **Sphingomyelins** are formed when the choline from a phosphatidylcholine is transferred to ceramide, leaving behind a diacylglycerol. **Glycolipids** are formed as UDG-glucose and UDP-galactose are added to ceramide. **Gangliosides** are just complex glycolipids that also contain sialic acids such as neuraminidic acid.

Sphingolipids are largely degraded within lysosomes by **sphingolipases** and **ceramidases**, while glycolipid side chains are first specifically degraded by a variety of saccharidases, including **β-galactosidases** and **hexosaminidases**. A variety of **sphingolipidoses** result from the improper targeting of lysosomal enzymes involved in the degradation of sphingolipids. All of these disorders are characterized by the accumulation of complex lipids containing ceramide within the cells (particularly neurons), leading to cell death. *Many of these lysosomal storage disorders are particularly prevalent in* **Ashkenazi Jews**.

The Sphingolipidoses and Sulfatidoses

Lipids are constantly being degraded and resynthesized in the body. This process is essential to ensure that oxidized and otherwise chemically altered lipids are removed from membranes and replaced with intact lipids. The sphingolipidoses and sulfatidoses are disorders of lipid degradation and are all recessive lysosomal storage disorders. Essential lysosomal enzymes involved in the degradation of particular lipids are mutated and individuals homozygous for these inactivating mutations accumulate those lipids within the lysosomes of particular organs of the body, resulting in the pathology of the disease. As these lipids accumulate, the cells in which they accumulate become dysfunctional. The sphingolipidoses are summarized in Table 2.2.

Tay-Sachs Disease Hexosaminidase A, a lysosomal enzyme involved in the degradation of ganglioside GM2, is mutated in this disease. GM2 ganglioside is normally present in the myelin sheaths of neurons, in the sarcolemma of cardiomyocytes, and in the membranes of hepatocytes. The myelin sheaths of neurons, formed by cells called oligodendroglia in the brain, are constantly being degraded and reformed. Without hexosaminidase A, damaged GM2 ganglioside accumulates in oligodendroglia, resulting in their death and eventually demyelination of neurons, resulting in their degeneration. Early symptoms of the disease develop by 6 months of age and are primarily due to this neurodegeneration. A normally developing infant ~6 months begins to deteriorate and lose both motor and intellectual capacity. The "cherry-red" spot on the macula (at the rear of the eye) is a classic feature of the disease and is due to neurodegeneration within the macula.

Table 2.2 The sphingolipidoses

Disease	Enzyme deficiency	Accumulating product	Important features	Treatment
Tay–Sachs	Hexosaminidase A	GM2 ganglioside (brain)	**Cherry red spot on macula**	None
			Mental retardation, blindness	
			Death by age 3	
			Ashkenazi-Jewish descent	
Gaucher	β-glucocerebrosidase	Glucocerebroside (brain, liver, spleen, bone marrow)	**Tissue paper macrophages**	Enzyme replacement therapy (imiglucerase)
				Glucosylceramide
				Synthase inhibitors
Niemann–Pick	Sphingomyelinase	Sphingomyelin	**Cherry red spot on macula**	Glucosylceramide
			Mental retardation	Synthase inhibitors
			Hepatosplenomegaly	
			Death by age 3	
Krabbe	Galactocerebrosidase	Galactocerebroside	**Multinucleated globoid cells**	Bone marrow transplant

(continued)

Table 2.2 (continued)

Disease	Enzyme deficiency	Accumulating product	Important features	Treatment
Fabry	α-galactocerebrosidase A	Ceramide trihexoside (systemic endothelial cells)	**Angiokeratomas**	Enzyme replacement therapy (agalsidase)
			Renal failure, corneal clouding	
			X-linked recessive	
Metachromatic leukodystrophy	Arylsulfatase A	Sulfatide (brain, kidney, liver, nerves)	Cerebral palsy	None
			Mental retardation	
			Seizures, blindness	
Farber	Acid ceramidase	Ceramide (brain, liver, joints, soft tissues)	Mental retardation	None
			Joint contractures, xanthomas	

Gaucher Disease Glucocerebroside accumulates in phagocytic cells throughout the body (spleen, liver, lungs, bone marrow) due to deficiency of the lysosomal enzyme glucocerebrosidase. Glucocerebroside is a component of the cell membranes of erythrocytes and leukocytes. All of these cells have a finite life span and are eventually phagocytosed by macrophages of the reticuloendothelial system, the body's housekeeping system involving the liver, spleen, and bone marrow. These macrophages normally degrade all of the components of the red and white blood cells, but without glucocerebrosidase, glucocerebroside accumulates within the lysosomes of these macrophages, leading to macrophage dysfunction. These abnormal macrophages resemble crumpled tissue paper histologically, leading to the pathognomonic for the disease, ***tissue paper macrophages***. These macrophages accumulate in bone marrow, spleen, and liver. Patients have anemia from bone marrow dysfunction, hepatosplenomegaly, and lung and kidney dysfunction.

Niemann–Pick Disease Sphingomyelin is an essential membrane lipid in the myelin sheaths of neurons and also within the plasma membranes of erythrocytes. Sphingomyelinase deficiency results in the accumulation of sphingomyelin in oligodendroglia within the brain and macrophages of the reticuloendothelial system. From this, you could expect that the symptoms of the disease may be a combination of those observed in Tay-Sachs disease and Gaucher disease. Indeed, this is the case, with infants developing neurological deficits similar to those present in Tay-Sachs disease by 6 months of age and later developing hepatosplenomegaly. As with Tay-Sachs disease, Niemann–Pick disease is associated with the cherry-red spot on the macula.

Krabbe Disease Deficiency of galactocerebrosidase leads to the accumulation of galactosylceramide, an essential component of myelin, within lysosomes in oligodendroglia, resulting in neurodegeneration in a mechanism similar to that observed in Tay-Sachs disease. A feature of this disease is that accumulating galactosylceramide also induces macrophages of the brain, called microglia, to form multinucleated giant cells, called ***globoid cells***. This is the histological pathognomonic of this disease. Early symptoms of the disease result from neurodegeneration with developmental delay, hypotonia, microcephaly, and absent reflexes. Eventually seizures develop, with death ensuing.

Fabry Disease Alpha-galactosidase A deficiency results in the accumulation of ceramide trihexoside primarily within endothelial cells, leading to compromised blood flow and the formation of abnormal capillaries called angiokeratomas. Compromised blood flow within the capillary beds of the kidney leads to renal failure, while angiokeratomas form in the skin and corneas, leading to corneal clouding.

Most of these can be treated with enzyme replacement therapy. Because cells are constantly endocytosing material from the extracellular space, it is possible to simply intravenously infuse a patient with functional enzyme. Because these lysosomal enzymes are normally functional only at the acidic pH of the lysosome, they are harmless in the blood and extracellular fluid. Once they are endocytosed, they end up in lysosomes of the cell, where they can be activated by the acidic pH and perform their degradative function.

There are two other major lysosomal storage disorders that are not defects in sphingolipid metabolism but rather defects in glycosaminoglycan metabolism, called mucopolysaccharidoses. These are **Hurler Syndrome** *and* **Hunter Syndrome**. *Hurler syndrome results from a deficiency in α-l-iduronidase. The disease is associated with corneal clouding and mental retardation. Hunter syndrome results from a deficiency in iduronate sulfatase and results in a milder form of disease associated with some mental retardation but no corneal clouding. Hunter syndrome is X-linked recessive.*

Eicosanoids

Eicosanoids are important signaling molecules derived from fatty acids. They act as **autacoids**, locally acting signaling mediators that generally act within the cell in which they are formed or rarely on adjacent cells. They are generally short lived. Many important drugs, including acetaminophen (Tylenol), aspirin, and non-steroidal anti-inflammatory drugs (NSAIDS) work by modulating enzymes involved in the production of eicosanoids. Eicosanoids found in the human body are derived primarily from eicosatetraenoic acid (arachidonic acid), but also eicosapentaenoic acid (EPA) and rarely eicosatrienoic acid (usually during states of deficiency in the essential fatty acids). Important prostanoids and their functions are presented in Table 2.3.

Arachidonic acid is found esterified to the SN2 position of phospholipids in the plasma membranes. **Phospholipase A_2 frees arachidonic acid by cleaving the ester linkage. This is the rate-limiting step for the synthesis of all eicosanoids!** Once arachidonic acid is freed, it is rapidly converted to one of a number of eicosanoids depending on the enzyme expression profile of the cell. The activity of phospholipase A_2 is upregulated by a number of inflammatory mediators, including TNF-α, IFN-γ, and others. The synthesis of the eicosanoids is shown in Fig. 2.17.

Prostanoids Formed by the cyclooxygenases (COX1 and COX2).

COX-1 is expressed in most tissues. It is described as a "housekeeping" enzyme, regulating normal cellular processes (such as gastric cytoprotection, vascular homeostasis, platelet aggregation, and kidney function) and is stimulated by hormones or growth factors. This is an essential function of various prostaglandins.

COX-2 is usually undetectable in most tissues; its expression is increased during states of inflammation, or experimentally in response to mitogenic stimuli. As an example, growth factors, phorbol esters, and interleukin-1 stimulate the expression of COX-2 in fibroblasts, while endotoxin serves the same function in monocytes/macrophages. COX-2 is constitutively expressed in the brain, kidney, bone, and probably in the female reproductive system.

Prostaglandins are largely vasodilators and bronchoconstricors, generally pro-inflammatory by initiating various cytokine cascades, inflammatory mediators, enhanced pain, and fever.

Table 2.3 The eicosanoids

Product	Location	Function
Prostaglandins		
PGE_2	Mast cells, macrophages, vascular smooth muscle, brain, kidney	Gastroprotection
		Diuresis
		Pain/hyperalgesia
		Vasodilator
		Immunomodulator
		Fever
PGF_2	Uterus, airways, vascular smooth muscle, eyes	Smooth muscle contraction (abortifacient at uterus)
		Bronchoconstrictor
PGD_2	Brain, mast cells, airways	Smooth muscle contraction
		Inhibits mast cell aggregation
PGI_2 (prostacyclin)	Endothelium, platelets, kidney, brain	Counteracts thromboxanes
		Vasodilation
		Inhibits platelet aggregation
TXA_2	Platelets, macrophages, vascular smooth muscle, kidneys	Vasoconstriction
		Platelet activation
		Bronchoconstriction
Leukotrienes		
LTB_4	Neutrophils	PMN activation (migration, degranulation, superoxide generation)
LTC_4, LTD_4, LTE_4 (cysteinyl leukotrienes)	Mast cells, eosinophils, basophils	Bronchoconstriction (main mediators in asthma)
		Vasoconstriction
		Reduce cardiac contractility
		Decrease coronary blood flow
Lipoxins		
LXA_4, LXB_4	Leukocytes	Vasodilation
		Block leukotriene function
Aspirin-triggered lipoxins (15 epimers)	PMN	Inhibit neutrophils
		Block cell proliferation

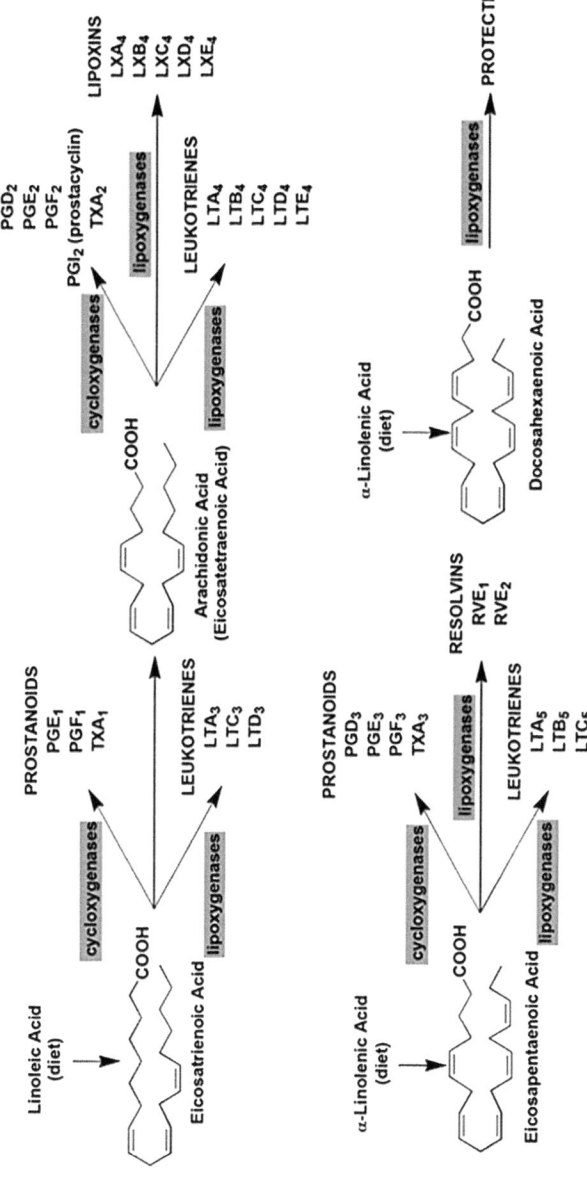

Fig. 2.17 The eicosanoids and their parent fatty acids

Prostaglandin E$_2$ (PGE$_2$): An important housekeeping prostaglanding involved in vasodilation, maintaining blood flow to the gastric mucosa (gastric protection) and renal cortex. Importantly, it is also a potent inflammatory mediator, leading to hyperalgesia (heightened sensation of pain) and fever. *A true double-edged sword!*

Prostacyclins (prostaglandin I$_2$—PGI$_2$) have the important and distinct effect of being anti-thrombotic.

Thromboxanes are largely vasoconstrictory and prothrombotic.

Lipoxygenase Pathway—synthesizes leukotrienes, lipoxins, resolvins, and protectins.

Leukotrienes—formed by the lipoxygenase pathway and are typically pro-inflammatory mediators. The common precursors to the leukotrienes are the hydroperoxyeicosatetraenoic acids (HPETEs).

Leukotriene B$_4$ (LTB$_4$)—primarily serves an immunomodulatory function.

Cysteinyl Leukotrienes (LTC$_4$, LTD$_4$, LTE$_4$)—important mediators of bronchoconstriction and allergic reactions such as **asthma** and **anaphylaxis.**

Lipoxins—formed by the lipoxygenase pathway and are typically anti-inflammatory mediators.

Resolvins—compounds derived from **eicosapentaenoic acid (EPA)** and act as potent anti-inflammatory molecules.

Protectins—compounds derived from **docosahexaenoic acid (DHA)**; immunomodulators.

Epoxins—formed by the epoxygenase pathway; important for regulation of blood flow and vascular tone in the kidney and other organs.

Isoprostanes Phospholipids containing arachidonic acid can be peroxidized as part of a natural oxidative process, especially during **oxidative stress**. When this oxidized phospholipid containing arachidonic acid is cleaved by phospholipase A_2 and processed in the cyclooxygenase, **isoprostanes** result. During oxidative stress, levels of isoprostanes in the blood are elevated. These compounds appear to activate a variety of oxidative stress response pathways.

Anandamide (*N*-arachidonylethanolamine): This is synthesized by **phospholipases** and is involved in **analgesia** and **pleasure sensing pathways**. It is an **endocannabinoid** and thus binds to the CB1 cannabinoid receptor. Cannabinoids contained in marijuana (*Cannabis sativa*) seem to co-opt the normal anandamide signaling pathways.

Essential Differences Among the Eicosanoid Families

Why does it matter that different fatty acid precursors can give different classes of eicosanoids? Depending on the number of double bonds, eicosanoids have very different activities. For example, the prothrombotic activity of TXA_2 is greater than the antithrombotic activity of PGI_2. Thus, when arachidonic acid is the major cellular precursor for prostaglandin synthesis, there is a tendency toward a prothrombotic state. Conversely, the prothrombotic activity of TXA_3 is much less than the antithrombotic activity of PGI_3. Thus, when eicosapentaenoic acid (EPA) is the major precursor for prostaglandin synthesis, there is a tendency toward an antithrombotic state. *** This may be the major mechanism by which fish oils (of which eicosapentaenoic acid and docosahexaenoic acid are the major constituents) improve cardiovascular health.*** We are only now beginning to understand the functional differences between the various classes of eicosanoids.

Additionally, **eicosapentaenoic acid (EPA)** and **docosahexaenoic acid (DHA)** give rise to resolvins and protectins, respectively, through the lipoxygenase pathway. These are the major ω-3 components of fish oils, and any commercial fish oil preparation will predominantly contain these two fatty acids.

The Dangers of COX-2 Selective Inhibition (The VIOXX Story) The cardiovascular risks of COX-2 inhibition seem largely to result from an ensuing imbalance between *prostacyclin* and *thromboxane* synthesis. COX-2 specifically initiates prostacyclin synthesis in the vascular endothelium. When COX-2 is inhibited, prostacyclin production drops dramatically. However, COX-2 seems less important in thromboxane production. Thus, the balance tips in the favor of thrombosis, leading to a prothrombotic state and vasoconstriction. The prothrombotic state leads to platelet aggregation and endothelial injury, while the vasoconstriction can lead to hypertension. Both of these are significantly increase the risk of adverse cardiovascular events. The reference to the paper that shows the role of COX-2 in prostacyclin production is given below, along with the abstract of the paper.

Conversely, the primary effect of NSAIDs (nonselective COX blockers) is to inhibit both COX-1 and COX-2, thereby impairing the ultimate transformation of arachidonic acid to prostaglandins, prostacyclin, and thromboxane. Thus, both thromboxanes and prostacyclins are downregulated simultaneously.

Metabolic Changes During Fasting

The immediate source of energy during the earliest stages of fasting is blood glucose. These stores are maintained up to approximately 12–18 h by hepatic glycogen reserves.

After approximately 12–18 h, hepatic glycogen stores are depleted. At this point, the liver undertakes gluconeogenesis. Specifically, fatty acid oxidation increases, producing acetyl-CoA. This serves as the primary source of ATP for gluconeogenesis. Amino acids derived from muscle breakdown serve as the primary substrates for gluconeogenesis, as will be described in the amino acid metabolism review.

Ketogenesis occurs simultaneously with gluconeogenesis in the early days of fasting. Some of the acetyl-CoA generated from fatty acid oxidation is metabolized in the TCA to yield ATP for gluconeogenesis, while the rest is used to form ketone bodies.

Over time, as protein reserves are depleted, usually within the first week of fasting, ketogenesis overtakes gluconeogenesis as the primary fuel generating pathway. However, some glucose is needed for proper brain function, so a basal level of gluconeogenesis is also maintained.

Cholesterol

Cholesterol is a multifunctional lipid that not plays an important role in regulating the rigidity of plasma membrane of all cells but also serves as a metabolic precursor to (1) bile acids; (2) steroid hormones, including mineralocorticoids, glucocorticoids, and sex hormones; and (3) vitamin D. The structure of cholesterol is given in Fig. 2.18.

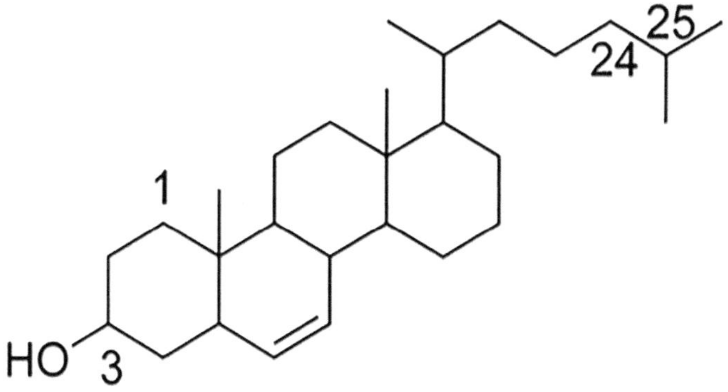

Fig. 2.18 Cholesterol

Cholesterol Biosynthesis

Cholesterol is derived both from the diet and from endogenous synthesis within the liver. The liver excretes approximately 1.2 g of cholesterol per day into the bile. In addition, the average American diet contains approximately 0.4 g of cholesterol. Thus, the major source of cholesterol in the intestine is the liver!

The general schema of cholesterol biosynthesis is given in Fig. 2.19. Acetyl-CoA is the major starting material for cholesterol biosynthesis. The synthesis of cholesterol can be divided into five phases: (1) the synthesis of mevalonate from acetyl-CoA; (2) the conversion of mevalonate to dimethylallyl pyrophosphate (DMAPP) and isopentenyl pyrophosphate (IPP); (3) the conversion of DMAPP and IPP into squalene (a 30 carbon chain); (4) the cyclization of squalene to produce a 30 carbon steroid known as **lanosterol**; (5) the conversion of lanosterol to cholesterol (a 27 carbon steroid) through the removal of 3 carbons. The first four phases occur in the cytosol, while the last step occurs in the endoplasmic reticulum. *Hence, cholesterol synthesis also relies on the citrate shuttle to produce cytosolic acetyl-CoA.*

The first phase of cholesterol synthesis is the most important in terms of regulation and pharmacological targeting and therefore is worthwhile knowing in detail and is presented on the next page. The first step is the formation of acetoacetyl-CoA from two acetyl-CoA molecules and is catalyzed by **thiolase**. The second stem is the formation of 3-hydroxy-3-methylglutaryl-CoA (HMG-COA) from acetoacetyl-CoA and acetyl-CoA. This is catalyzed by **HMG-CoA synthase**. The final step is the formation of mevalonate from HMG-CoA. This step requires **NADPH** and is catalyzed by ***HMG-CoA reductase***.

Cholesterol Biosynthesis

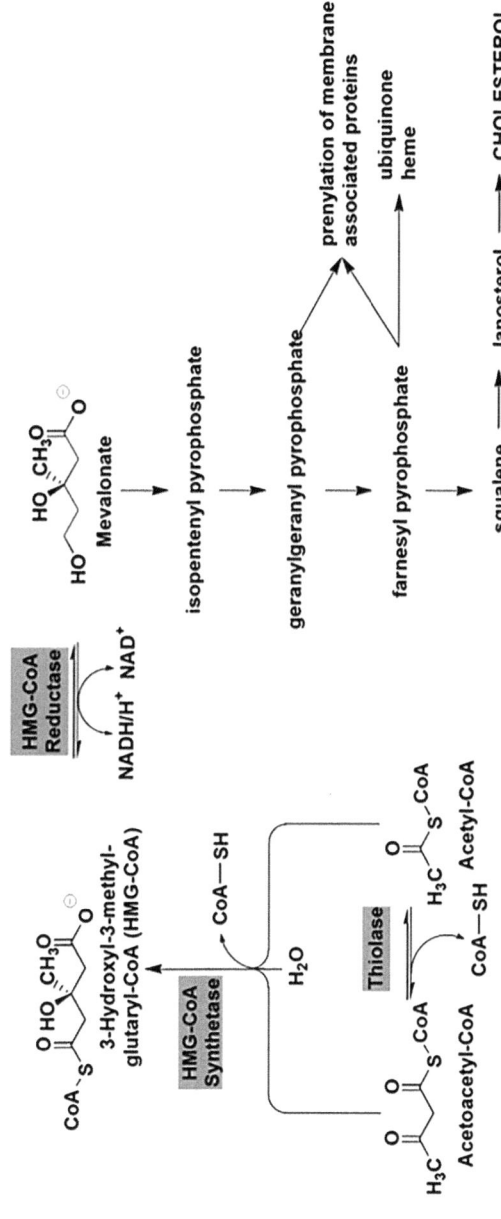

Fig. 2.19 Cholesterol biosynthesis

Regulation of HMG-CoA Reductase

This is the most regulated step of cholesterol synthesis. Again, there is a large degree of product inhibition. Cholesterol and bile acids inhibit HMG-CoA reductase transcription. In the absence of cholesterol and bile salts, sterol regulatory element binding protein (SREBP) translocates to the nucleus and activates HMG-CoA reductase transcription. In the presence of cholesterol and bile salts, SREBP is prevented from translocating to the nucleus, thus reducing HMG-CoA reductase transcription.

Mevalonate can also inhibit the enzyme allosterically. Insulin, glucagon, and other hormones also have important regulatory roles here. Insulin and thyroid hormone increase HMG-CoA reductase activity and thus stimulate cholesterol synthesis, while glucagon and glucocorticoids inhibit HMG-CoA reductase activity and thus inhibit cholesterol synthesis. These are presented in the following.

The powerful cholesterol reducing drugs known as ***statins*** are HMG-CoA reductase inhibitors. While statins have other atheroprotective activities, including the induction of **Klf-2** expression, their major mode of cholesterol reduction is reducing endogenous cholesterol biosynthesis by inhibiting HMG-CoA.

Notice at this point that insulin and glucagon regulate carbohydrate metabolism, fatty acid metabolism, and cholesterol metabolism. It should now become apparent that these are hormones that regulate metabolism in response to the overall nutritional state of the body (fed vs. fasting) and regulate all the metabolic processes in conjunction. Thus, diseases such as <u>diabetes mellitus</u> are truly <u>pan-metabolic diseases</u>, not just diseases of carbohydrate metabolism!

The other phases are worthwhile knowing in as much detail as I have given in Fig. 2.19, although there is much more available in the larger literature for those who are interested.

Lipid Transport

Lipids are insoluble or sparingly soluble in the serum and thus require highly sophisticated transport mechanisms that prevent their precipitation within blood vessels. The lipoprotein system transports triglycerides and cholesterol throughout the body for use by the tissues and/or storage. We can divide lipoprotein pathways into those that are primarily involved in triglyceride transport and those that are involved in cholesterol transport, although this is an extremely imperfect division.

Lipoproteins classically have two components:

- Hydrophilic shell: Apolipoproteins, phospholipids, unesterified cholesterol.
- Hydrophobic core: Triacylglycerol and cholesterol esters.

Apolipoproteins

AI—activates LCAT.
B-48—catalyzes the formation of chylomicrons.
B-100—catalyzes the formation of VLDL particles.
CII—activates the enzyme lipoprotein lipase.
E—induces lipoprotein uptake by the liver.

Chylomicrons

Chylomicrons are the first system that is important in the transport of intestinally absorbed long chain fatty acids and cholesterol. Medium chain fatty acids are generally soluble and enter portal blood directly to be metabolized at the liver. Cholesterol is absorbed through a channel known as **NPC1L1** in enterocytes. This cholesterol is then largely esterified to **cholesteryl esters** by **acyl-Coa:cholesterol acyltransferase** (**ACAT**). Long chain fatty acids are generally absorbed directly through the plasma membrane in their **uncharged** form. In the intestinal epithelial cells (enterocytes), these fatty acids are then converted back to triglycerides by **diacylglycerol acyltransferase** (**DGAT**).

In the enterocytes, the ApoB gene is transcribed. The mRNA for ApoB is then edited by **ApoB Editing Complex 1** (**APOBEC1**), a protein which converts a glutamate codon to a stop codon. This results in the synthesis of **ApoB-48** in the enterocyte, a protein that is **48%** of the length of the full length protein.

Within the **endoplasmic reticulum**, Apo B-48 is **translipidated** by **microsomal transfer protein**, which basically adds triglycerides and cholesterol to Apo B-48. Thus, the **chylomicron** is formed. Chylomicrons are secreted into the interstitial fluid from the basolateral membrane of enterocytes. They are too large to enter the capillaries, so instead they are taken up by **lymphatics** and delivered to the blood through the **thoracic duct** (now you know why the **cisterna chyli** is known by that name).

Once in the blood, the main function of chylomicrons is to deliver triglycerides to tissue. This process is shown in Fig. 2.19. At this point chylomicrons are inactive. They must be **activated** by gaining a molecule of **Apo CII** from circulating HDL particles, which act as reservoirs of this apolipoprotein. Once they gain Apo CII, chylomicrons are activated and can deliver their lipids to tissues.

Muscle and adipose tissue produce a protein called **lipoprotein lipase (LPL)**. They secrete this protein, which binds to glycoproteins on endothelial cells. Thus, endothelial cells lining capillaries in muscle and adipose tissue selectively possess this protein. LPL hydrolyzes triglycerides in the core of chylomicrons to produce free fatty acids. These free fatty acids then get absorbed directly through the plasma membrane of the local cells. These chylomicrons shrink as their fatty acids are slowly removed. These chylomicrons then interact with HDL once again, now exchanging **Apo CII** and getting **Apo E**, becoming **chylomicron remnants**.

Chylomicron remnants are important in the process of **reverse cholesterol transport**, which will be described subsequently. Apo E binds to the **LDL receptor** or the **LDL-receptor Related Protein (LRP)**, and these particles are then endocytosed by the liver, thus completing the life cycle of the chylomicron.

Summary of Chylomicrons

- Least dense of lipoproteins.
- Formed in smooth ER of intestinal mucosa and secreted into lymphatics to transport dietary lipids.
- Triacylglycerol in the chylomicrons is hydrolyzed by lipoprotein lipase in vasculature of cardiac, skeletal muscle, and adipose tissue.

- Apo B48 is unique to chylomicrons.
- Apo CII activates lipoprotein lipase and results in FA release to the heart, skeletal muscle, and mammary glands.
- Apo E allows clearance of chylomicron remnants by the liver.

VLDL, IDL, and LDL

As you remember, there are two sources of cholesterol and triglycerides—the diet and the liver! Hence there are two modes of delivery. As the chylomicron is the delivery system for lipids absorbed through the diet, the **VLDL** system is the mode of systemic delivery for lipids synthesized by the liver. The pathways for the two systems are remarkably similar, but different in some very critical ways! The majority of the cholesterol in the body is synthesized in the liver—this far outweighs the amount of cholesterol received through the diet!

In the liver, hepatocytes do not possess the APOBEC1 editing machinery and thus synthesize **Apo B-100**, the full length Apo B protein. This is then translipidated by MTP in the liver to form VLDL. The liver then secretes VLDL particles into the blood for peripheral delivery of triglycerides. This may have evolved as a system to ensure sufficient peripheral delivery of fatty acids when there is insufficient dietary intake.

Once in the periphery VLDL must be activated just like chylomicrons. This process is shown in Fig. 2.20. VLDL particles get Apo CII from HDL particles, after which they can be metabolized by peripheral LPL. Eventually, as these particles shrink, about 50% of these particles exchange Apo CII and get Apo E from HDL, thus becoming **VLDL remnants**. These VLDL also participate in **reverse cholesterol transport** and eventually, 50% are taken up by the LDL receptor and metabolized by the liver just like chylomicrons.

However, the other 50% of VLDL is not taken up by the liver. Instead it continues to be metabolized by LPL and become **intermediate-density lipoproteins** (**IDL**). A portion of these IDL particles are then taken up by the LDL receptor, which binds

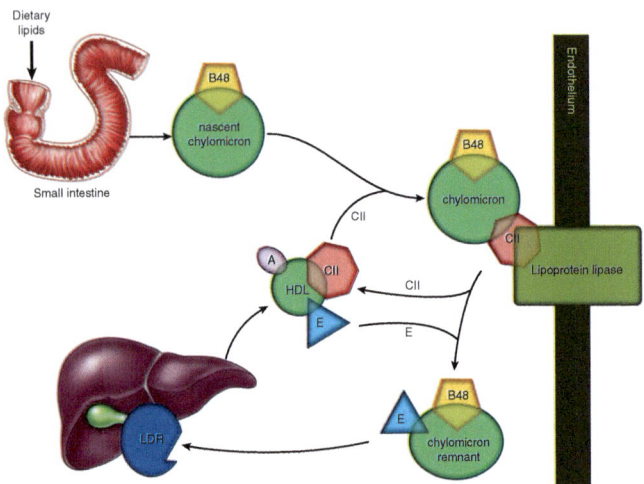

Fig. 2.20 The chylomicron cycle

the Apo E on IDL, and thus are metabolized just like VLDL remnants and chylomicron remnants.

The remaining portion of this IDL is metabolized by **hepatic lipase** to **low-density lipoproteins (LDL)**. Importantly, LDL particles lose their affinity for Apo E and thus lose it to HDL particles. *Thus, LDL particles do not have Apo E. Hence they do not bind well to the LDL receptor! This is a very important point— LDL particles do not bind well to the LDL receptor!!!* Thus, they cannot be taken up by the liver with any great efficiency. Weak interactions of Apo B-100 with the LDL receptor allow its clearance after an extended circulatory lifetime.

Thus, LDL is (1) very rich in cholesterol because most of the fatty acids have been removed by the lipases and (2) cannot be efficiently cleared from the blood. Thus, these cholesterol rich particles float in the blood for extended periods of time, during which time they can be oxidized, glycosylated, or otherwise altered. This modified LDL binds **scavenger receptors** on macrophages in the blood vessels and is then internalized. These macrophages are converted to **foam cells** as they continue to take up modified LDL particles. These foam cells secrete a variety of cytokines and chemokines that cause localized inflammation and thus contribute to **atherogenesis** and **atherosclerosis**.

VLDL Summary

- Made in the liver to transport TG and CE.
- More enriched in CE than chylomicrons.
- Also metabolized by lipoprotein lipase to produce IDL remnants.

LDL Summary

- Generated from VLDL and IDL by further action of hepatic lipase.
- Increased proportion of cholesterol esters in the core.
- Transport cholesterol to extrahepatic tissue.
- Retain only apo B100—interacts with LDL receptor on tissue for endocytosis.

HDL and Reverse Cholesterol Transport

HDL serves two major functions: (1) to act as an apolipoprotein reservoir, holding the exchangeable apolipoproteins Apo CII, Apo E, and others; and (2) to transport excess cholesterol from the periphery back to the liver for excretion. This second process is referred to as **reverse cholesterol transport** and is shown in Fig. 2.21.

In HDL formation, the first step is the secretion of **Apo AI**. This apolipoprotein is then translipidated by **ABCA1**, a protein located in the sinusoids of the liver, and thus the **nascent HDL particle** is generated. This particle then becomes mature HDL. HDL accepts cholesterol from peripheral tissues, which accumulates on its surface. The Apo AI activates

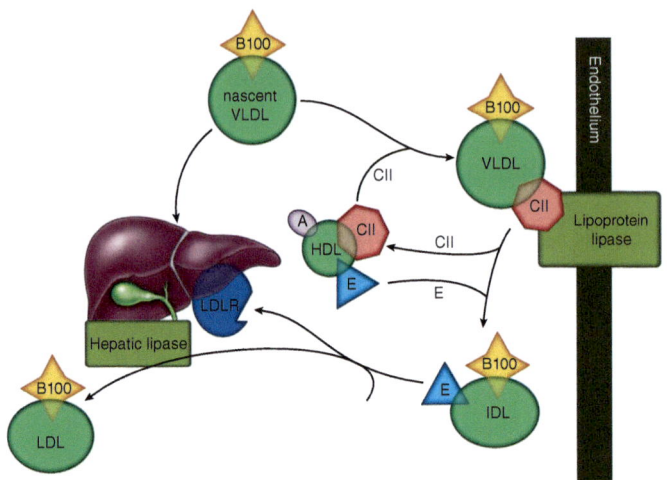

Fig. 2.21 The VLDL cycle

lecithin:cholesterol acyltransferase (LCAT), which esterifies this cholesterol so that cholesterol does not accumulate on the surface of HDL. This is essentially a flux generating reaction that allows for more cholesterol to then be added to the surface of the HDL particle.

Thus, the HDL particle accumulates cholesterol primarily in the form of **cholesteryl esters**. This is where **chylomicron remnants** and **VLDL remnants** come into play. Remember that these particles are traveling back to the liver for uptake by hepatocytes. **Cholesterol Ester Transfer Protein (CETP)** transfers these cholesteryl esters from HDL to the remnant particles.

Two important points about CETP: (1) By transferring cholesteryl esters from HDL to remnants, it is reducing HDL cholesterol (i.e., it is reducing the total amount of blood cholesterol that is in the form of HDL). (2) By removing cholesteryl esters from HDL, it is extending the life of the HDL particle such that it can absorb more cholesterol from peripheral tissues. Thus, CETP is actually

Disorders of Lipid Transport

extending the usable life of the HDL particle by allowing for cholesterol to be transported back in particles that will anyway be metabolized. *What does this mean about CETP inhibitors?*

Once the HDL particle has enlarged to a critical size, it binds to **hepatic scavenger receptors** and is taken up to be metabolized in the liver, thus completing the cycle of reverse cholesterol transport.

HDL Summary

- Synthesized by the liver.
- Approximately 50% protein.
- Core region relatively empty when secreted by the liver.
- Serve as a circulating reservoir for apoproteins.
- Move cholesterol from extrahepatic tissue to the liver.
- Lecithin cholesterol acyltransferase (LCAT) is a plasma enzyme that esterifies HDL cholesterol.

Other Lipoproteins of Note

These have significant cardiovascular risk, although their exact functions remain obscure.

Lipoprotein (a) or **Lp(a)**—pronounced LP-little-a.

Lipoprotein X.

Disorders of Lipid Transport

Both hyperapolipoprotenemias and hypolipoproteinemias cause disease in humans, as shown in Table 2.4.

Table 2.4 Common (and commonly tested) disorders of lipid transport

Disease	Defect	Lipid profile	Important features
Familial hypercholesterolemia (type IIa)	LDL receptor deficiency	Heterozygotes: LDL ~300	Achilles tendon xanthomas
		Homozygotes can have LDL >900	Premature atherosclerosis
			Xanthelasma palpebrarum
Familial defective ApoB	ApoB gene mutation resulting in defective binding of ApoB100 to the LDL receptor	Elevated LDL	Similar features to familial Hypercholesterolemia
Chylomicronemia (type I hyperlipoproteinemia)	Lipoprotein lipase deficiency	Elevated triglycerides	Cutaneous xanthomas
			Elevated risk of pancreatitis
LCAT deficiency	LCAT deficiency	Decreased HDL	Corneal opacification
			Hemolytic anemia
Tangier disease	ABCA1 deficiency	Significantly decreased HDL	Tonsillar xanthelasma (yellow tonsils)
		Elevated triglycerides	Hepatosplenomegaly
			Neuropathy
CETP deficiency	CETP deficiency	Increased HDL	Juvenile corneal opacifications
			Lipomatosis (multiple lipomas)

Familial combined hyperlipidemia	Undetermined gene (possibly Apo CII); autosomal dominant	Elevated LDL, triglycerides	Premature atherosclerosis
Polygenic hypercholesterolemia	Undetermined defects	Decreased HDL Increased total cholesterol, LDL	Premature atherosclerosis
Familial hypertriglyceridemia	Undetermined defect	Elevated triglycerides, VLDL	Elevated risk of pancreatitis
Polygenic low HDL	Undetermined defect	Low HDL	Premature atherosclerosis
	Associated with lack of exercise, diabetes mellitus, and carbohydrate-rich diet		

Lipid-Lowering Drugs

Statins (atorvastatin, simvastatin, rosuvastatin, lovastatin, pravastatin) are **competitive inhibitors** of **HMG-CoA Reductase**, the rate-limiting step in cholesterol synthesis. This ultimately reduces the production of cholesterol in the liver. The liver in turn "senses" low cholesterol since there is decreased production and a compensatory increase in LDL receptor trafficking to liver surface is seen, leading to increased VLDL, IDL, and LDL uptake and decreased circulating LDL. *Thus, the key point to understand here is that statins increase LDL uptake by the liver by decreasing endogenous hepatic cholesterol synthesis.* This is the key mechanism by which statins work. Statins also target Klf-2, which may be another atheroprotective target.

Bile acid resins (cholestyramine, colesevelam, colestipol) **block enterohepatic circulation** by binding up bile acids in the intestine. This increases the liver's metabolism of cholesterol to bile acids, thus reducing the overall cholesterol levels. They primarily reduce LDL levels but have little to no effect on HDL levels.

Fibrates (gemfibrozil, clofibrate) **activate PPARα**, causing increased expression of lipoprotein lipase. This in turn increases triacylglycerol removal from circulation. How exactly this reduces cholesterol levels is still uncertain, although as we have discussed, circulating fats, especially saturated fats, have potent effects in increasing serum cholesterol levels.

Very High Dose Niacin (1500–3000 mg/day) decreases LDL by inhibiting VLDL production and also increases HDL, possibly by increasing the half-life of Apo AI. This is the only existing drug that increases HDL by any appreciable amount.

Cholesterol absorption inhibitors (Ezetimibe) block cholesterol absorption in the intestine through the NPC1-L1 channel in enterocytes, thus increasing the excretion of cholesterol in the stool.

CETP inhibitors (Torcetrapib) were tried because CETP deficiency leads to increased HDL, as summarized in Table 2.4. However, they actually increased mortality and were abandoned.

Theoretically, while they may have increased the total cholesterol found in HDL, they actually inhibited the overall process of reverse cholesterol transport!

Clinical Aspects of Cholesterol Homeostasis

Atherosclerosis is the primary result of the accumulation of oxidized cholesterol within the vascular tunica **intima**. This is usually caused by deranged **LDL** metabolism, and the **LDL:HDL ratio** is a good clinical predictive parameter of cardiovascular risk.

A Model of Atherogenesis

1. Excess LDL in bloodstream forms concentration gradient → begins to accumulate in intima of artery wall.
2. LDL is modified (oxidized, etc.) within intima, but process still unclear—have no idea whether cause or effect.
3. Modified LDL chemotactic for monocytes/macrophages.
4. Modified LDL taken into macrophages through constitutively expressed scavenger receptors → foam cells.
5. Efflux of lipid from foam cells can be controlled through ABC transporter expression.
6. Smooth muscle proliferation and "inflammation" due via foam cell and endothelial signaling → atherosclerotic plaque.

Dietary Influences Increased intake of polyunsaturated fatty acids and monounsaturated fatty acids and reduced intake of saturated fatty acids and trans fatty acids seems to reduce the **LDL:HDL ratio** and result in reduced cardiovascular risk.

Lifestyle Influences Smoking, obesity, and hypertension seem to generally increase serum cholesterol levels, while exercise and weight loss may reduce these levels.

Cholesterol Metabolism

Cholesterol is converted to a number of metabolites, including bile acids, steroid hormones, and vitamin D.

Bile Acids

Bile acids are emulsifying agents that aid in the absorption of fats in the intestine and are synthesized from cholesterol through hydroxylation. Importantly, once bile acids are formed from cholesterol, cholesterol cannot be regenerated. The key enzyme in this process is **7α-hydroxylase**, the rate-limiting step in bile acid formation. This process relies on **NADPH**, **Vitamin C**, and **molecular O_2**. Once formed, bile acids are released in bile to emulsify dietary lipids. Bile acids are then reabsorbed in the ileum and recycled in a process known as enterohepatic circulation, which reduces the need for constant hepatic synthesis of bile acids.

Steroids

A **hormone** is a substance which exerts its effect at a location distant from its synthesis. Steroid hormones are by definition lipids and thus readily cross the cell membrane. The main action of steroid hormones is to induce or repress the expression of specific genes which, in turn, alter cell function. Once steroids cross the cell membrane, they bind to protein receptors in the cytosol and activate these receptors. Steroid-bound activated receptors then translocate to the nucleus, where they bind to DNA and alter gene expression.

Steroid hormones are synthesized primarily in the adrenal cortex, although the ovaries are important sources of estrogens and progesterone and the testes are important sources of testosterone. The adrenal gland is divided into three zones, the zona glomerulosa, the zona fasciculata, and the zona reticularis, respectively, layered from the surface of the cortex to the center. The core of the adrenal gland is the medulla, which is involved in catecholamine synthesis, which is covered in Chap. 3.

The zona glomerulosa is responsible for the synthesis of aldosterone, a mineralocorticoid involved in sodium and water homeostasis that acts primarily on the kidney. The zona fasciculate is responsible for the synthesis of cortisol, a glucocorticoid responsible for the regulation of stress responses, including increasing blood glucose concentrations and modulation immune response. The zona reticularis is responsible for synthesizing adrenal androgens. While the functions of each of these hormones are generally taught in endocrine pathophysiology, the synthesis of these hormones is schematized in Fig. 2.22.

All of the adrenocortical enzymes are part of the P450 cytochrome oxidase family of enzymes and also have corresponding P450 classification names. <u>Desmolase</u> is considered the rate-limiting enzyme of steroid synthesis.

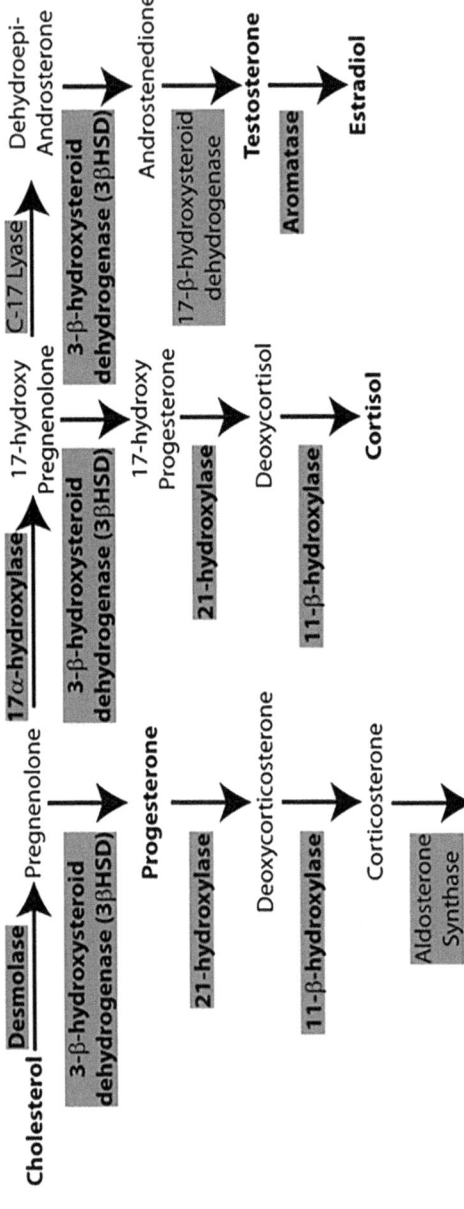

Fig. 2.22 Enzymes involved in the synthesis of steroid hormones

Congenital Adrenal Hyperplasia

Enzyme deficiencies can cause inability to produce certain hormones and accumulation of precursor molecules or shunting to other pathways. The adrenal gland is over-stimulated and thus hypertrophies due to lack of the normal negative feedback cycle. There are several types:

Lipoid congenital adrenal hyperplasia—results from the failure to metabolize cholesterol resulting from **desmolase deficiency**. The adrenals fill with cholesterol globules, hence the name lipoid CAH. There is a severe deficiency of all steroid hormones, and males are severely **undervirilized**, being raised as infertile females in most cases. There is also marked **salt wasting** due to the lack of mineralocorticoids.

3β-hydroxysteroid dehydrogenase deficiency—as expected from the above pathway, also results in severe deficiency of all steroid hormones. The symptoms are essentially identical to those of lipoid CAH.

17α-hydroxylase deficiency—inability to produce the glucocorticoids and sex steroids results in shunting to the mineralocorticoid pathway, leading to **salt retention**, which causes **hypertension** (as you will learn in HST 110: Renal Pathophysiology). Again, males are severely **undervirilized**.

21-hydroxylase deficiency—inability to produce glucocorticoids or mineralocorticoids, leading to **salt wasting1**. Shunting to the sex steroid pathway leads to overproduction of adrenal androgens, leading to **virilization** in females.

11β-hydroxylase deficiency—as with 21-hydroxylase deficiency, **virilization** in females is the most common symptom.

Androgens

Testosterone is synthesized in Leydig cells of testes in a process similar to that of adrenal steroid synthesis. Dihydroxytestosterone (DHT), a more potent androgen, is produced from testosterone by 5alpha-reductase, an enzyme found in peripheral tissues.

Female Sex Hormones

Progesterone produced by corpus luteum within the ovary and the placenta. *Estradiol* is converted from testosterone by the enzyme aromatase, found in the granulosa cells of the ovary. Testosterone in turn is produced by the theca cells of the ovary.

Vitamin D

Vitamin D biosynthesis involves four distinct steps, depicted in Fig. 2.23. (1) The liver converts cholesterol to 7-dehydrocholesterol. (2) Then ultraviolet radiation incident on

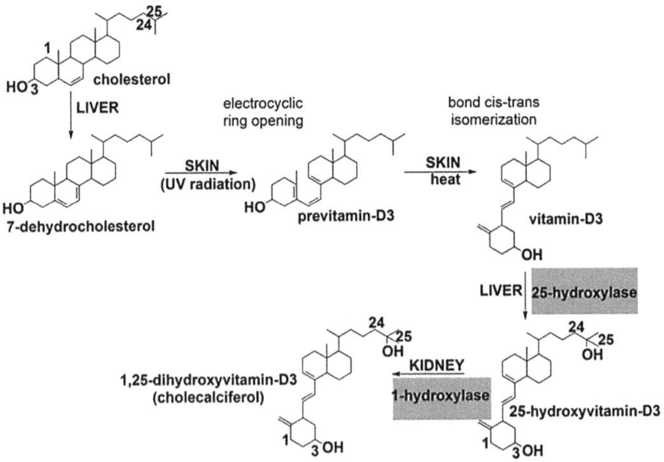

Fig. 2.23 Vitamin D synthesis

the **skin** catalyzes an electrocyclic ring opening to produce previtamin D_3. This is then isomerized to vitamin D_3 (**ergocalciferol**) at body temperature spontaneously. (3) Vitamin D_3 is converted to 25-hydroxyvitamin D_3 in the **liver** by **25-hydroxylase**. (4) 25-Hydroxyvitamin D_3 is then converted in the **kidney** by **1-α-hydroxylase** to **1,25-dihydroxyvitamin D_3** (**calcitriol**), the active form of vitamin D. Vitamin D_2 (**ergocalciferol**) can be derived from the diet from plant sources and can also be converted to 25-hydroxyvitamin D_2 in the liver and then to 1,25-dihydroxyvitamin D_2 in the kidney.

Vitamin D deficiency leads to rickets in children and osteomalacia in adults. Both of these diseases are characterized by continued formation of the bony collagen matrix, but insufficient mineralization, ultimately leading to soft bones. Primary causes of vitamin D deficiency include nutritional deficiency (extremely common in the USA—up to 80–90% of the population currently) and decreased sun exposure. Deficiencies in cortisol, the active form, can result from renal failure.

Important Diseases of Lipid Metabolism

Major Metabolic Diseases

Atherosclerosis LDL accumulation in macrophages within blood vessel walls leading to the formation of atherosclerotic plaques that compromise blood flow through (1) constriction of flow, (2) acute thrombotic occlusion, and (3) distal embolization with occlusion, leading to end organ hypoperfusion, causing myocardial infarctions and strokes. **Diabetic Ketoacidosis:** Absolute insulin deficiency results in the unabated oxidation of fatty acids in the liver and production of ketones, leading to acidosis. Concomitant unabated gluconeogenesis results in hyperglycemia. This is in effect the opposite of the fasting hypoketotic hypoglycemia state.

Disorders of Lipid Transport (Table 2.4)

Some Important Enzyme Deficiencies in Carbohydrate Metabolism

Fasting Hypoketotic Hypoglycemia (carnitine deficiency, carnitine palmitoyltransferase I mutations, medium chain acyl-CoA dehydrogenase (MCAD) deficiency)—inability to produce ketone bodies in hypoglycemic states propionic acidemia—results in hyperammonemia and encephalopathy.

Methylmalonic acidemia—results in hyperammonemia and encephalopathy X-Linked adrenoleukodystrophy—results in progressive brain damage and adrenal gland dysfunction Zellweger syndrome—results in liver failure, mental retardation, and seizures.

The sphingolipidoses (Table 2.1).

The congenital adrenal hyperplasias.

Amino Acid Metabolism 3

Biologically Important Amino Acids

All natural amino acids (except glycine which is achiral) are **L-amino acids** (they rotate plane-polarized light counterclockwise). They all have the same relative stereochemical configuration (as shown in Fig. 3.1) at the central carbon, known as the α-carbon. Amino acids exist as a **zwitterion** (doubly charged neutral species) at physiological pH. This is because the carboxylic acid has a pK_a less than the physiological pH and the **protonated amine** has a pK_a greater than the physiological pH.

There are 20 major amino acids that are utilized in human metabolism. The 20 amino acids can be further classified as nutritionally essential or nutritionally nonessential amino acids. **The Nutritionally Essential Amino Acids** are amino acids the liver cannot synthesize and thus ones that humans must obtain from their diets. These include histidine (H), isoleucine (I), leucine (L), lysine (K), methionine (M), phenylalanine (F), threonine (T), tryptophan (W), and valine (V). **A good mnemonic for these is**

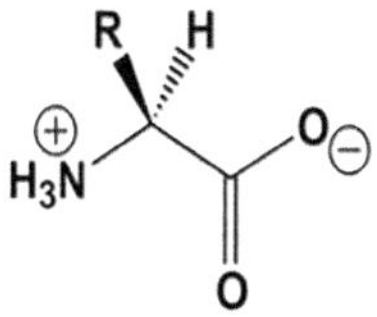

Fig. 3.1 Amino acid structure

V. Yanamadala, *Essential Medical Biochemistry and Metabolic Disease*, https://doi.org/10.1007/978-3-031-59394-9_3

PVT. TIM HiLL or PVT. TIM HALL (because arginine is essential in infancy). The Nutritionally Nonessential Amino Acids are ones that the liver can synthesize and include glutamate (E), glutamine (Q), alanine (A), asparagine (N), aspartate (D), cysteine (C), glycine (G), proline (P), serine (S), tyrosine (Y), and arginine (R).

Kwashiorkor is a disease that results when a child is weaned onto a starchy diet poor in protein. Symptoms result from protein deficiency and include skin lesions, edema (with significant abdominal distension), anemia, and steatosis (fatty liver). The typical clinical picture is a young child with a swollen belly. *FYI: Kwashiorkor literally means first-second, meaning a disease that is seen in the first child when the second child is born because the first child is weaned from his mother's milk (a protein rich source) to a carbohydrate-rich diet.*

Marasmus is a disease that results from general caloric deficiency, which includes protein deficiency. Symptoms include tissue and muscle wasting, loss of subcutaneous fat, and edema. This is also known as protein-calorie malnutrition. Serum albumin is frequently low in marasmic individuals because the liver is unable to synthesize adequate albumin given the protein deficit.

Amino acids are further classified by the nature of their R group as shown in Fig. 3.1 as acidic, basic, neutral, or hydrophobic. The chemical nature of the R group determines the function of that amino acid within a protein. Frequently, a single mutation in a protein that changes one amino acid to another results in complete alteration of the function of that protein and causes human disease. Acidic amino acids are ones that become negatively charged at blood pH and include aspartate and glutamate. Basic amino acids are ones that accept a proton and become positively charged at blood pH and include lysine, arginine, and histidine. Neutral amino acids are hydrophilic amino acids that remain neutral at blood pH and include serine, threonine, and cysteine. Hydrophobic amino acids can be further classified as aliphatic, including glycine, alanine, valine, leucine, isoleucine, and proline, and aromatic, including phenylalanine, tyrosine, and tryptophan.

Overview of Amino Acid Metabolism

Proteins ingested in the diet are broken down by proteases secreted by the stomach (pepsin) and pancreas (trypsin, chymotrypsin, etc.). These proteases cleave peptide bonds that link amino acids together, thus releasing small peptides containing short chains of amino acids. These peptides are further broken down by peptidases produced by enterocytes within the small intestine lumen. This process is discussed in detail in gastrointestinal pathophysiology courses and thus only cursorily covered here. Free amino acids are then absorbed through the small intestine in much the same way that free sugars are, as discussed in Chap. 1. Uptake of amino acids is mediated by Na^+-amino acid symporters. Intracellular Na^+ concentrations are kept low by the action of the Na^+/K^+-ATPase, and this Na^+ gradient drives the cotransport of Na^+ and amino acids. Amino acids then exit enterocytes into the blood down their concentration gradient through facilitated diffusion through amino acid channels on the basolateral membranes. Amino acids are then utilized in protein synthesis and can ultimately be degraded.

Biosynthesis of the Nutritionally Nonessential Amino Acids

Most of these synthetic reactions are one step—you may be happy to know. The majority of this synthesis occurs in the liver for systemic delivery of amino acids, although particular reactions occur in other tissues. For example, the brain is a major site of glutamate and glutamine synthesis.

Most of these reactions are catalyzed by aminotransferases, which interconvert α-keto acids and amino acids in a process catalyzed by pyridoxal phosphate (PLP), a metabolite of **Vitamin B6 (pyridoxine)**. The chemistry of pyridoxal phosphate is given in more detail in Appendix 1. Some of these α-keto acid and amino acid interconversions are shown below, examples of these reactions are shown subsequently.

α-keto acids	Amino acids
α-ketoglutarate	Glutamate
Oxaloacetate	Aspartate
Pyruvate	Alanine
Glyoxylate	Glycine

Glutamate is synthesized from α-ketoglutarate, an intermediate of the TCA, by **glutamate dehydrogenase**, which requires NADPH and PLP, or by **glutamate synthase**, which requires $FADH_2$ and PLP, as shown in Fig. 3.2.

Glutamine is synthesized from glutamate by **glutamine synthase** in an ATP dependent manner, as shown in Fig. 3.3. **Note that this is an irreversible reaction.**

Asparagine is synthesized from aspartate by **asparagine synthase** in an ATP dependent manner that is very similar to the mechanism above for glutamine synthase and is shown in Fig. 3.4. The only difference is that **the source of ammonia is not free ammonium but rather glutamine, which is converted to glutamate**.

Alanine is synthesized directly from pyruvate by **alanine aminotransferase (ALT)**, also known as **serum glutamate pyruvate**

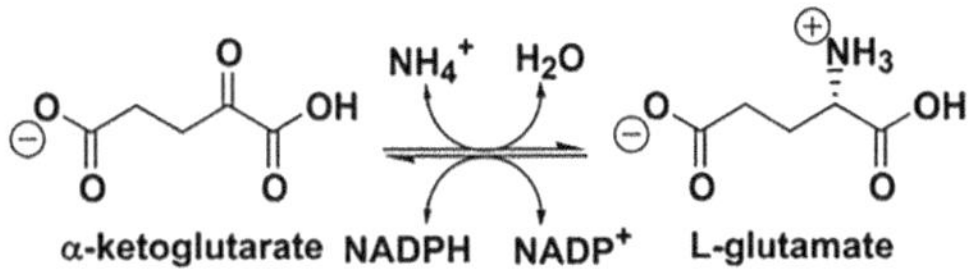

Fig. 3.2 Glutamate synthesis

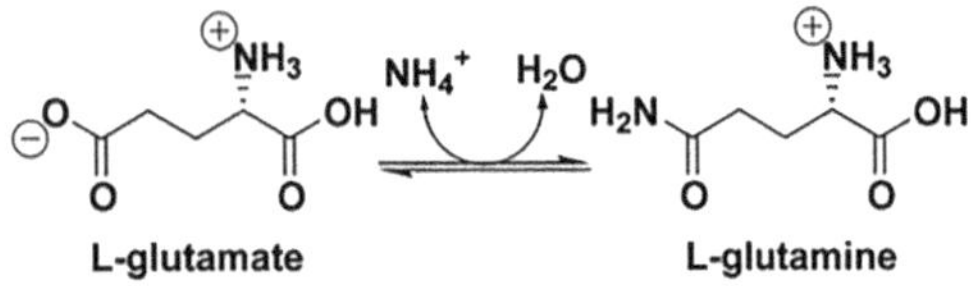

Fig. 3.3 Glutamine synthesis

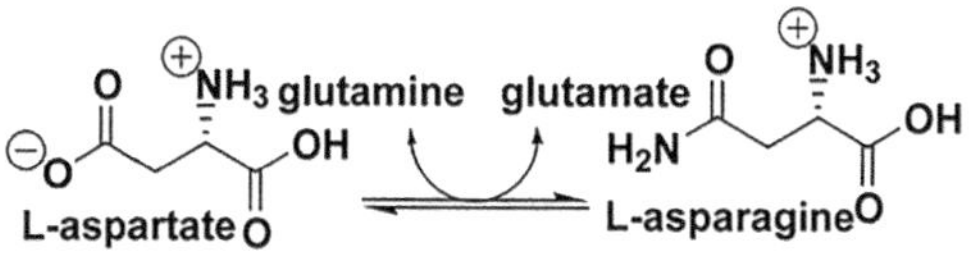

Biosynthesis of the Nutritionally Nonessential Amino Acids

Fig. 3.4 Asparagine synthesis

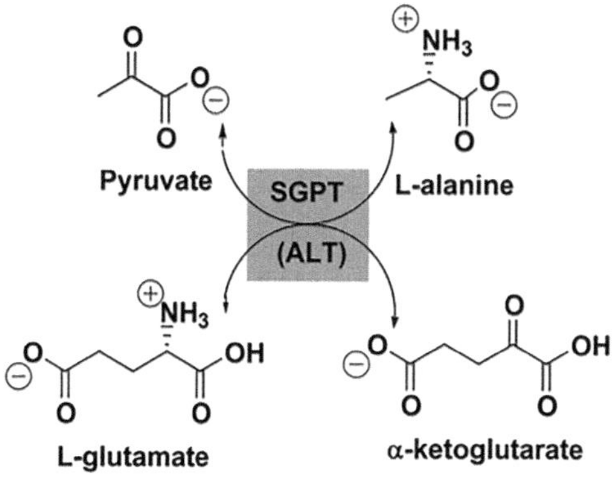

Fig. 3.5 Alanine synthesis by serum glutamic pyruvic transaminase (SGPT), also known as alanine transaminase (ALT)

transaminase (SGPT)—you should know both names. This is a slightly more complicated reaction, called a **transamination** as implied by the name, and is shown in Fig. 3.5. The amino group from glutamate is transferred to pyruvate, in the process producing α-ketoglutarate and alanine. The reverse can also occur. This enzyme requires **pyridoxal phosphate (PLP)**, a metabolite of **Vitamin B6 (pyridoxine)**, as an essential cofactor. *This is an enzyme that is measured in the blood as a liver function test (LFT). Elevated ALT levels suggest liver dysfunction that can be caused by a multitude of etiologies.*

Aspartate is generated from oxaloacetate. Just as the transamination of pyruvate yields alanine, the transamination of oxaloacetate (another TCA intermediate) yields aspartate. Hence, just replace pyruvate with oxaloacetate and alanine with aspartate in the ALT reaction (Fig. 3.5)! This reaction is catalyzed by **aspar-

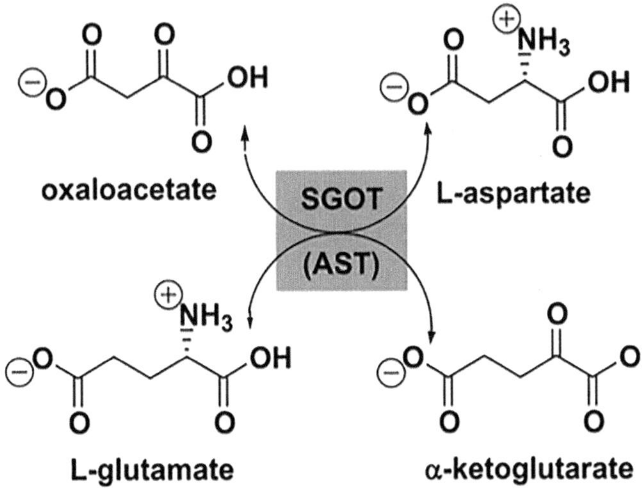

Fig. 3.6 Aspartate synthesis by serum glutamic oxaloacetic transaminase (SGOT), also known as aspartate transaminase (AST)

tate aminotransferase (AST), also known as **serum glutamate oxaloacetate transaminase (SGOT)** and is explicitly shown in Fig. 3.6. This enzyme requires **pyridoxal phosphate (PLP)**, a metabolite of **Vitamin B6 (pyridoxine)**, as an essential cofactor. *AST is another enzyme that is measured in the blood as a liver function test (LFT). Elevated AST levels also suggest liver dysfunction that can be caused by a multitude of etiologies. ALT and AST are differentially elevated by various causes of liver dysfunction and are used clinically to further establish a differential diagnosis for liver failure, as you will learn in your gastrointestinal pathophysiology courses.*

Serine is synthesized from **3-phosphoglycerate** (a glycolysis intermediate) by a serine transaminase. **Glycine** can in turn be synthesized from **serine**, as shown in Fig. 3.7, by **serine hydroxymethyltransferase**, in a reaction that requires **folic acid** in the form of tetrahydrofolate. The biochemistry of folic acid and its derivatives is discussed in detail in Appendix 1. Alternatively, glycine can also be synthesized from **choline**.

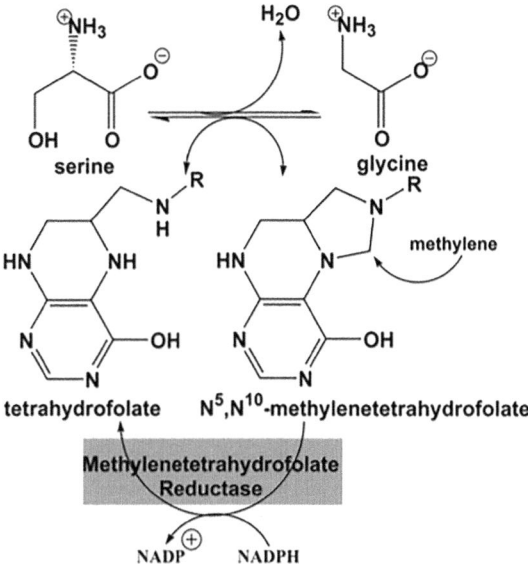

Fig. 3.7 Glycine synthesis from serine

Proline is synthesized from **glutamate** in an oxidative cyclization.

Cysteine is synthesized from **methionine** and **serine** in a reaction sequence that you should study carefully and is illustrated in Fig. 3.8. Methionine is first converted to S-adenosylmethionine (SAM) by S-adenosylmethionine synthase. SAM is an important methyl donor in a number of biochemical reactions in which it is ultimately converted to S-adenosylhomocysteine. **Methionine synthase** is one such enzyme that requires folic acid in the form of tetrahydrofolate (THF) as a cofactor and vitamin B12 as a regenerator of THF. Again, the chemistry of folic acid and its derivatives is discussed in detail in Appendix 1. The S-adenosylhomocysteine thus produced is hydrolyzed by S-adenosylhomocysteine hydrolase to homocysteine and adenosine. Homocysteine is then condensed with serine to form cystathionine by **Cystathionine β-synthase**. Cystathionine then undergoes cleavage to form cysteine and α-ketobutyrate, a byproduct that enters the propionic acid pathway.

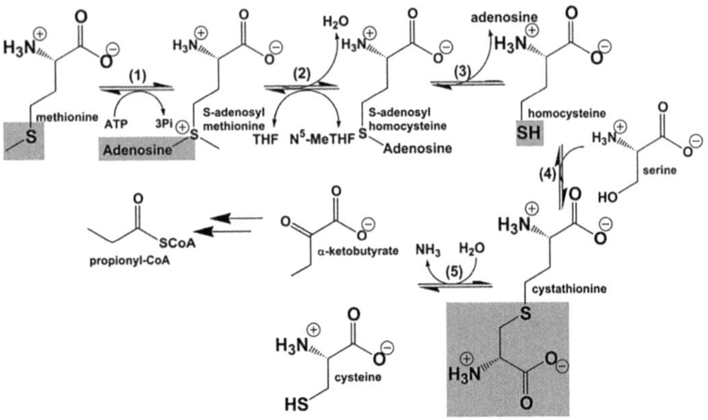

Fig. 3.8 Cysteine is synthesized from methionine in a five step process. Methionine is first converted to S-adenosylmethionine (SAM) by SAM synthase (1). SAM is then demethylated by Methionine Synthase (2) and other cellular enzymes that use SAM as a methylation cofactor, producing S-adenosylho-mocysteine. S-adenosylhomocysteine is then hydrolyzed to homocysteine by S-adenosylhomocysteine hydrolase (3). Homocysteine and Serine are then combined by Cystathionine Synthase (4) to form Cystathionine, which is then hydrolyzed (5) to form cysteine and α-ketobutyrate, which is metabolized to propionyl-CoA. Propionyl-CoA is further metabolized as shown in Fig. 2.11

Mutations of cystathionine β-synthase are the most common cause of homocysteinuria. Mutations of methionine synthase are also known to cause homocysteinuria. Homocysteinuria is associated with mental retardation, premature atherosclerosis, premature osteoporosis, and other skeletal abnormalities, and ectopia lentis (displacement of the lens of the eye). The only available treatment is the limitation of methionine intake, and cysteine becomes an essential amino acid because it cannot be synthesized in this way.

Importantly, homocysteine levels are also elevated in both vitamin B12 and folate deficiencies because both of these factors are required for the conversion of homocysteine back to methionine. Homocysteine levels are frequently measured to assess the possibility of B12 and folate deficiency. The association of homocysteine with premature atherosclerosis is one which is being actively

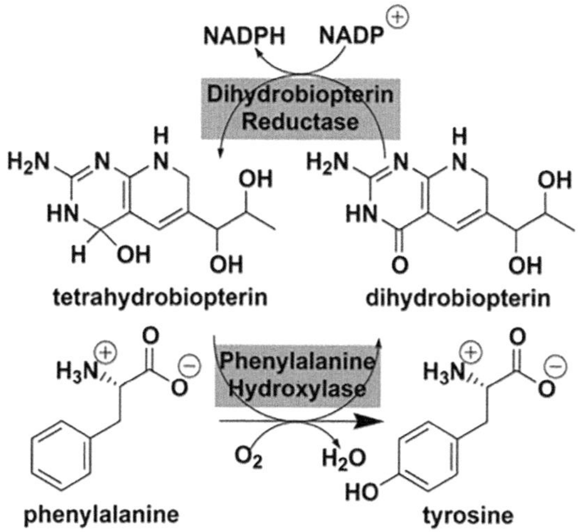

Biosynthesis of the Nutritionally Nonessential Amino Acids

Fig. 3.9 Tyrosine is synthesized from phenylalanine by phenylalanine hydroxylase, the enzyme that is mutated in phenylketonuria

investigated. Homocysteine appears to cause vascular injury by promoting intimal thickening, elastic lamina disruption, smooth muscle hypertrophy, marked platelet accumulation, and the formation of platelet-enriched occlusive thrombi.

Tyrosine is synthesized from **phenylalanine** by **phenylalanine hydroxylase** in a reaction that requires **tetrahydrobiopterin**, **NADPH**, and molecular oxygen, as illustrated in Fig. 3.9. This enzyme hydroxylates phenylalanine using molecular oxygen, and *mutation of this enzyme leads to phenylketonuria*. In phenylketonuria, accumulating phenylalanine and its metabolites such as phenylpyruvate cause **mental retardation**, **growth retardation**, **fair skin** (due to lack of tyrosine, and thus melanin), and **eczema**. The body has a **musty odor** because phenylalanine and its metabolites, being aromatic compounds, have a strong odor. **Tyrosine becomes an essential amino acid**, because it can no longer be synthesized from phenylalanine. The treatment is to **limit phenylalanine intake** (including such sources as **NutraSweet**) and the **supplement tyrosine**.

The other hyperphenylalaninemias (type II–V) are defects in tetrahydrobiopterin metabolism. A deficiency in biopterin itself, or in dihydrobiopterin reductase (type II hyperphenylalaninemia), the enzyme that converts dihydrobiopterin back to tetrahydrobiopterin in and NADPH dependent manner, or in other enzymes involved in biopterin synthesis (dihydrobiopterin synthase), can also result in a phenylketonuria like syndrome.

Arginine—synthesized in the **urea cycle**, as will be described subsequently.

Important Amino Acid Derivatives

Amino acids give rise to many important hormones **Amino Acid Derivatives**, small molecule catalysts, and signaling compounds in the body.

Histamine is derived from histidine through decarboxylation. It stimulates dilation of arterioles and post-capillary venules, contraction of veins, and contraction of endothelial cells, all in preparation for infiltration of immunological cells.

S-Adenosylmethionine (SAM) is derived from methionine **Amino Acid Derivatives** and ATP. This is the cellular methylating agent and the synthesis of SAM was shown as part of the cysteine synthesis pathway earlier in Fig. 3.8.

Thyroxine (thyroid hormone) is derived from free radical dimerization of two **tyrosines** followed by iodine electrophilic aromatic substitution. Just know that it is derived from tyrosine for now. You will learn the details of its synthesis in HST 060: Endocrinology.

Tyrosine, tryptophan, and glutamate are important sources of **neurotransmitters**. The **tyrosine-derived neurotransmitters** include **dopamine, norepinephrine, epinephrine**, the synthesis of which is shown in Fig. 3.10. The **rate-limiting step** is **tyrosine hydroxylase**. **Tryptophan-derived neurotransmitters** include **serotonin (5-hydroxytryptamine, 5-HT)** and **melatonin**. This synthesis is remarkably similar to the one for tyrosine-derived neurotransmitters. Serotonin is derived from tryptophan by hydroxylation by **tryptophan hydroxylation**, the **rate-limiting**

Important Amino Acid Derivatives

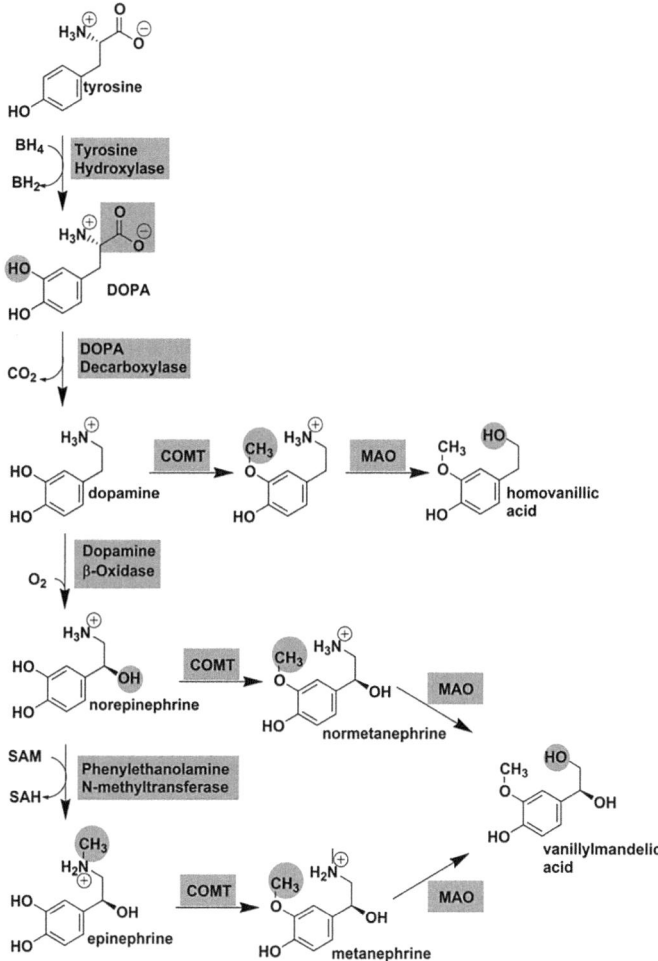

Fig. 3.10 The synthesis and degradation of important tyrosine-derived neurotransmitters

step, followed by decarboxylation. Melatonin is derived from serotonin by acetylation and methylation. The **glutamate-derived neurotransmitters** include **glutamate** itself and **γ-aminobutyric acid (GABA)**. GABA is synthesized from glutamate by **gluta-**

mate decarboxylase, an enzyme that requires **pyridoxal phosphate** Amino Acid Derivatives.

The tyrosine-derived neurotransmitters are eventually degraded by monoamine oxidase (MAO) and catechol-O-methyltransferase (COMT). COMT converts epinephrine to metanephrine and norepinephrine to normetanephrine. Both metanephrine and normetanephrine in turn are converted to vanillylmandelic acid by MAO. Dopamine is converted to homovanillic acid by the action of each enzyme successively in a similar fashion. These processes are also shown in Fig. 3.10.

Creatine, an important store of high-energy phosphate equivalents in muscle, is derived from **arginine**. Creatine is subsequently metabolized to creatinine, which is excreted by the kidney. Blood creatinine levels are measured as a way to assess kidney function.

Melanin is derived from **tyrosine** and is synthesized in melanocytes, which are neural crest derived cells. The key enzyme is **tyrosinase**, and deficiencies in this enzyme can cause **albinism**.

Nitric Oxide is generated from **arginine** by **nitric oxide synthase (NOS)**.

Taurine, a major component of bile, is synthesized from cysteine as part of the cysteine degradation pathway.

Porphyrin (discussed at the end of the review sheet) is generated from **glycine**.

The Essence of Protein Synthesis

Proteins are synthesized on ribosomes (located either free in the cytosol or associated with rough endoplasmic reticulum) based on an mRNA template using tRNAs that are conjugated to individual amino acids. Proteins are frequently folded with the assistance of molecular chaperones. This topic is usually covered in molecular biology as thus only mentioned briefly here.

Protein Degradation

There are two pathways for degradation: **lysosomal degradation** and **proteasomal degradation**.

The lysosome primarily degrades membrane and endocytosed proteins using **acid hydrolases** and **proteases**. This process is known as **autophagy** and appears to be primarily induced during starvation states to provide amino acids for gluconeogenesis when other stores are depleted. In autophagy, vesicles are formed around cellular organelles by secondary membranes, and these vesicles then fuse with lysosomes, where the contents are then degraded.

The **proteasome** is largely responsible for degradation of cytosolic proteins, including misfolded proteins and proteins whose expression must be downregulated. Proteins that are degraded by the proteasome must be **polyubiquitinated**. **Ubiquitin** is an 8.5kD protein that is conjugated to **lysine** residues on the protein to be degraded in an ATP dependent manner by **ubiquitin ligases**, **E1**, **E2**, and **E3**. In this reaction, ubiquitin is first transferred to **E1 ligase** (also known as the ubiquitin activating protein). Then **E2 ligase** (also known as the ubiquitin transfer protein) accepts ubiquitin from E1 ligase. **E3 ligase** (also known as the ubiquitin ligase) then catalyzes the transfer of the ubiquitin from E2 to a **lysine** on the target protein. This cycle is repeated to polyubiquitinate the target protein. Proteins targeted for degradation may be polyubiquitinated on one or several lysine residues. This process is demonstrated in Fig. 3.11.

The proteasome is a large polyprotein that consists of two caps and a core. The caps have rings of 6-ATPases that unfold the protein to allow entry into the core. The core proteasome has four subunit rings (2 outer α rings that play a structural role and 2 β rings that are the catalytic parts). This structure is shown in Fig. 3.12. Each β ring has six catalytic sites, which are known by their respective activity. The two trypsin-like sites cleave peptides

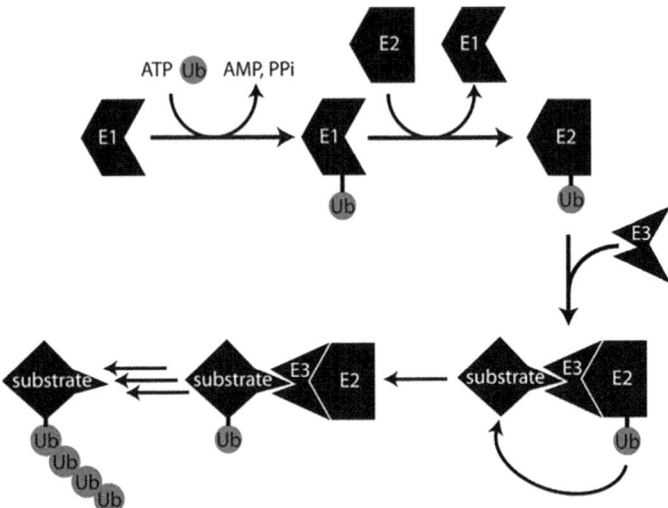

Fig. 3.11 Ubiquitination of a protein. E1 Ligase is first ubiquitinated (Ub) in a process that requires ATP. This Ub is then transferred to E2 Ligase. E3 Ligase then catalyzes the addition of this Ub to a substrate protein. Reiteration of this process leads to polyubiquitination of the substrate protein

after basic residues, the two chymotrypsin-like sites cleave peptides after hydrophobic residues, and the two caspase-like sites cleave after aspartate residues. The resulting small peptides are then released into the cytosol, where cellular proteases further break them down into amino acids. There are now a number of proteasome inhibitors in clinical trials for multiple myeloma and other cancers.

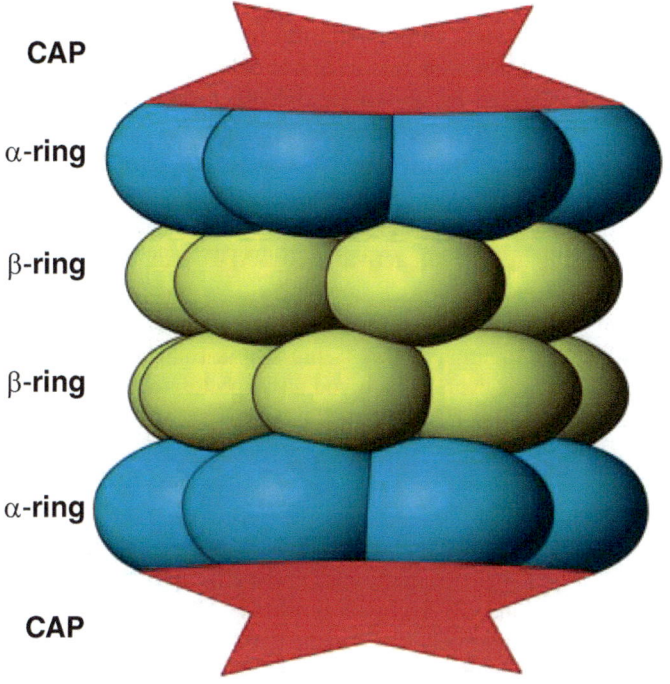

Fig. 3.12 The proteasome

Amino Acid Degradation

Amino acids are first typically degraded through **transamination** reactions, as mentioned earlier. This usually yields a metabolite that can directly feed either into glycolysis or the TCA. The amine nitrogen is carried by **glutamate** or **glutamine** and then converted to urea through the urea cycle for excretion in the urine.

The first step, **transamination**, is catalyzed by **transaminases**. For example, **alanine transaminase (ALT)** catalyzes the conversion of alanine and α-ketoglutarate to pyruvate and glutamate. This is the reverse reaction of alanine synthesis, shown in Fig. 3.5. Other amino acids are similarly transaminated. All aminotransferases require the cofactor **pyridoxal phosphate (PLP)**, which is derived from **vitamin B6 (pyridoxine)**.

The second step is the release of free ammonia from glutamate, which is catalyzed by **glutamate dehydrogenase**, in a reaction that is exactly the reversal of glutamate synthesis from α-ketoglutarate, or from glutamine, which is catalyzed by **glutaminase**, an enzyme that carries out the reverse reaction of glutamine synthase shown in Fig. 3.3. Glutamate dehydrogenase is allosterically regulated, **activated by ADP,** and **inhibited by GTP**.

The third step is the conversion of this ammonia, which is highly toxic, to urea, which is much less toxic. This is done through the urea cycle, which you are expected to know in great detail.

The Urea Cycle

The urea cycle has two purposes: (1) **the elimination of nitrogenous wastes** and (2) **arginine synthesis**. There are five major reactions that ultimately catalyze the formation of urea and fumarate from CO_2, ammonia, and aspartate. Fumarate in turn is converted to oxaloacetate through the TCA, and oxaloacetate is converted back to aspartate by AST. This secondary cycle is known as the aspartate-arginosuccinate shunt and prevents feedback inhibition through the accumulation of fumarate. *In adult humans, these reactions only take place in the liver. Importantly, for the fetus, the placenta plays many of the same roles as the liver in adults, including carrying out the urea cycle.* A schematic of the urea cycle and its auxiliary aspartate-arginosuccinate shunt is presented in Fig. 3.13.

Step I: Carbamoyl Phosphate Synthesis—Carbamoyl phosphate synthase I (CPSI) catalyzes the formation of **carbamoyl phosphate** from CO_2, NH_3, and ATP. This reaction also requires one molecule of ATP to provide the driving force, thus requiring a total of two ATP. This is the **rate-limiting step** of

The Urea Cycle

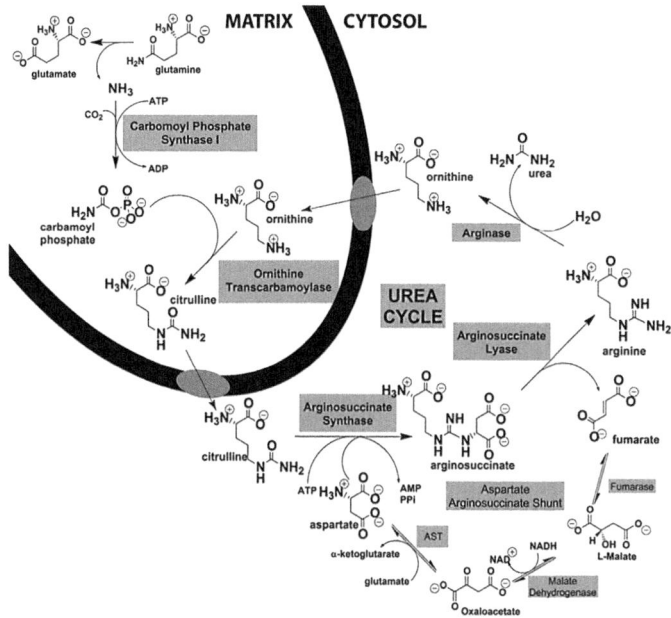

Fig. 3.13 The urea cycle. Within the mitochondrial matrix, ammonia released from glutamine is transformed to carbamoyl phosphate by the enzyme carbamoyl phosphate synthase I. Ornithine Transcarbamoylase then combines carbamoyl phosphate with orinithine to form citrulline. Citrulline then exits the mitochondrion to the cytosol, where it is combined with aspartate by arginosuccinate synthase to form arginosuccinate. Arginosuccinate lyase then releases fumarate to form arginine. Arginase then hydrolyzes arginine to urea and ornithine. Ornithine is recycled back into the mitochondrial matrix by the ornithine transporter ORNT1. Fumarate produced by arginosuccinate lyase is converted back to aspartate through the aspartate-arginosuccinate shunt, which utilizes enzymes of the Krebs Cycle, as shown in the bottom right hand corner

the urea cycle and takes place in the **mitochondrial matrix**. The NH_3 used in this process is generated from glutamine or glutamate as described earlier.

Step II: Citrulline Synthesis—Ornithine Transcarbamoylase catalyzes the formation of **citrulline** from **ornithine** and **carbamoyl phosphate** within the **mitochondrial matrix**. In the process, free phosphate is released.

Step III: Arginosuccinate Synthesis—**Arginosuccinate Synthase** catalyzes the formation of **arginosuccinate** from **aspartate** and **citrulline** in the **cytosol**. This process requires ATP and releases AMP and pyrophosphate.

Step IV: Arginine Synthesis—**Arginosuccinase** (**Arginosuccinate Lyase**) catalyzes the breakdown of **arginosuccinate** into **arginine** and **fumarate** (which enters the TCA) in the **cytosol**. This reaction is important for endogenous arginine synthesis.

Step V: Urea Synthesis—**Arginase** catalyzes the formation of **urea** and **ornithine** from **arginine**, thus completing the cycle. Ornithine passes back into the mitochondrion through the **ornithine transporter**.

An important part of understanding the urea cycle is accounting for the sources of nitrogen. The first nitrogen is delivered by glutamine, which releases a molecule of NH_3 that is used by CPSI. The second molecule of NH_3 is brought by aspartate that is used in step 3 by arginosuccinate synthase.

Regulation of the Urea Cycle

As you now know, ammonia is highly toxic to the body. Hence, carefully regulated nitrogen balance is essential for life. The urea cycle is regulated through (1) feed-forward regulation by ammonia, (2) hormonal regulation, and (3) allosteric regulation by N-acetylglutamate and alanine. Ammonia is known to induce the expression of urea cycle enzymes as a mechanism of feed-forward regulation. Glucagon also induces the expression of urea cycle enzymes as the urea cycle is essential for the disposal of nitrogen generated by the breakdown of amino acids used for gluconeogenesis.

Finally, carbamoyl phosphate synthase I is the rate-limiting enzyme in the urea cycle, as mentioned above, and hence it is highly regulated. *__It is allosterically activated by N-acetylglutamate__*. N-acetylglutamate in turn is formed from **acetyl-CoA** and **glutamate** in the liver by **N-acetylglutamate**

The Urea Cycle

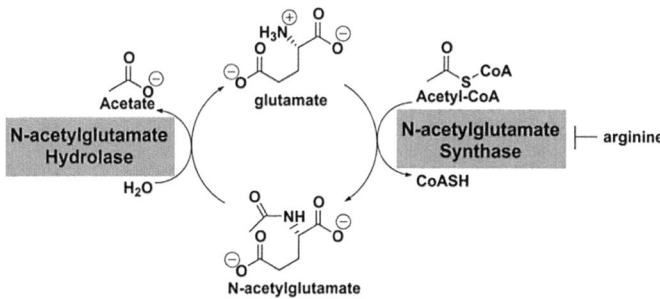

Fig. 3.14 The synthesis and degradation of N-acetylglutamate, an important regulator of the urea cycle enzyme CPS I

synthase, a reaction shown in Fig. 3.14. Hence, N-acetylglutamate senses both energy (acetyl-CoA) and the presence of amino acids (glutamate) in that when both of these are simultaneously high, N-acetylglutamate levels will also be high. *Hence, the urea cycle is upregulated when the levels of amino acids and overall energy stores are high, as immediately after a meal.* N-acetylglutamate synthase is also regulated by arginine by acting as an allosteric activator.

Hepatic Encephalopathy

Dysfunction of the brain is known as encephalopathy, and one cause is liver failure. As you probably now appreciate, the liver is a key metabolic organ. In liver failure, toxins normally metabolized by the liver accumulate in the blood, causing the brain and other organs to dysfunction. Hepatic encephalopathy is characterized by seizures, motor dysfunction, personality changes, mood changes, and even cognitive dysfunction (delirium). It is known to be caused by the effects of various toxins on neurons in the brain. Ammonia is one of these toxins that is known to cause neuronal swelling and dysfunction. Ammonia accumulates in the blood during liver failure because the urea cycle is non-functioning. Ammonia levels are frequently measured in cases of liver failure to determine whether or not treatment is succeeding. While the correlation between ammonia levels and symptoms of hepatic encephalopathy is currently a hotly debated topic with no clear consensus, measuring blood ammonia levels is something you will commonly see when you are on the wards.

Urea cycle defects occur in 1 per 70,000 live births, usually as a result of single base pair substitutions in one of the urea cycle enzymes. **All of these disorders are associated with hyperammonemia**. Most of these disorders present at birth or in early infancy except for arginase deficiency. CPSI deficiency is the most severe and is also known as **Hyperammonemia Type I**. OTC deficiency, also known as **Hyperammonemia Type II**, is the most common disorder and is X-linked. AS deficiency is rare. AL deficiency presents very early and is quite severe, while arginase deficiency is less severe and usually presents around 2–4 years of age. Defects in the ornithine transporter (ORTN1) lead to the **Hyperornithinemia, Hyperammonemia, and Homocitrullinuria Syndrome (HHH)**.

Treatment of these disorders involves

1. Reducing protein intake (hard to achieve especially in infants), thus reducing the need to metabolize the excess amino acids.
2. Hemodialysis to remove excess ammonia in patients with severe hyperammonemia.
3. Nitrogen scavenging drugs
   (a) Phenylacetate—complexes with glutamine to form phenylacetylglutamine, which can be excreted without being reabsorbed by the kidney
   (b) Sodium benzoate—complexes with glycine to form hippurate, which can be excreted without being reabsorbed by the kidney.
4. Reducing the amount of ammonia produced in the gut by bacteria, which have urease and thus catabolize whatever urea is present in the intestines to ammonia and thus adding to the total body ammonia pool. Antibiotics (such as neomycin) can help reduce the amount of ammonia produced by bacteria in the gut by simply reducing their numbers.

5. Trapping the ammonia that is produced in the gut by acidifying the large intestine and converting it to ammonium, which does not pass freely through cell membranes. Lactulose is a sugar that is not metabolizable by small intestine enzymes, but is metabolizable by bacteria in the large intestine. Metabolism of this sugar through glycolysis acidifies the large intestine, converting ammonia to ammonium ion, and trapping it in the feces.
6. Liver transplant—the ultimate cure in serious cases.

Arginine usually becomes an essential amino acid in patients with urea cycle defects—this is an important nutritional consideration.

Ammonia Transport: The Glutamine Cycle

Because ammonia is highly toxic, peripherally generated ammonia must be transported to the liver via a safe transporter. The major mechanism for doing this is **the glutamine cycle**. In **the glutamine cycle**, free ammonia is used to synthesize glutamine from glutamate by **glutamine synthase**. Note that this is an irreversible reaction that uses ATP. Glutamine then circulates in the blood. In the liver, glutamine is then converted back to glutamate by **glutaminase**, which releases free ammonia for use in the urea cycle. This is shown in Fig. 3.15.

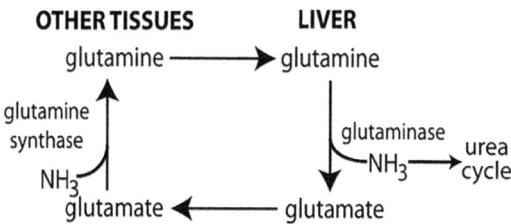

Fig. 3.15 The glutamine cycle

The Alanine Cycle

Amino acids derived from protein degradation in the muscle are converted to α-keto acids, which are substrates for glycolysis and the TCA, as described below in the section on catabolism of carbon skeletons. In turn, the amine group from that amino acid is transferred to pyruvate to produce alanine through transamination. Alanine then diffuses into the blood and then to the liver, where it is converted back to pyruvate for gluconeogenesis by **alanine aminotransferase**. The ammonia from glutamate eventually makes it to the urea cycle. **This is the primary way by which muscle protein is used for gluconeogenesis in the liver—free amino acids are used to produce alanine, which then makes it back to the liver for gluconeogenesis. This glucose can then be used by extrahepatic tissues.** The alanine cycle is shown in Fig. 3.16.

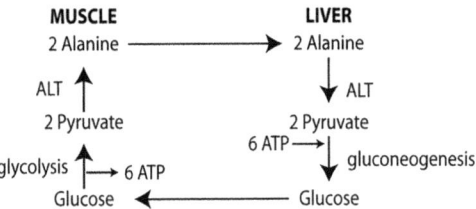

Fig. 3.16 The alanine cycle

Catabolism of the Carbon Skeletons

Once the amino acids are transaminated, they yield various metabolites that can then be further metabolized by the cell. Amino acids are divided into two classes, **glucogenic amino acids** and **ketogenic amino acids**, based on what products their metabolism yield. Glucogenic amino acids can be converted to glucose, whereas ketogenic amino acids are primarily converted to acetyl-CoA and then to ketone bodies. The only purely ketogenic amino acids are **leucine** and **lysine**. Four amino acids, **isoleucine**, **phenylalanine**, **tyrosine**, and **tryptophan**, are capable of contributing to both ketogenesis and gluconeogenesis. All other amino acids contribute predominantly to gluconeogenesis and are hence called glucogenic. This is summarized in Fig. 3.17.

To remind you, the **aspartate-arginosuccinate shunt**, shown in Fig. 3.13, interconnects the urea cycle and the TCA. Fumarate produced by arginosuccinate lyase in the urea cycle enters the TCA, where it is eventually converted to oxaloacetate. Oxaloacetate in turn is converted to aspartate by aspartate synthase, and this aspartate then is used by arginosuccinate synthase in the urea cycle. This shunt prevents the accumulation of byproducts of the urea cycle, which can act as feedback inhibitors and prevent the efficient disposal of ammonia.

Metabolic defects in the various catabolism pathways lead to a number of amino acid inborn errors of metabolism. Hence it is worthwhile to examine a few key catabolic pathways and learn the key enzymes whose mutation leads to prominent disease.

Glycine is transaminated to glyoxylate, the α-keto acid form of glycine, by **glyoxylate reductase/hydroxypyruvate reductase (GRHPR)**, an enzyme that co-converts alanine to pyruvate. This is a similar reaction to the ALT enzyme, using glycine in place of glutamate. Deficiencies in this enzyme result in **primary hyperoxaluria**, associated with the formation of calcium oxalate kidney stones (nephrolithiasis) as well as nephrocalcinosis, leading to renal failure and hypertension.

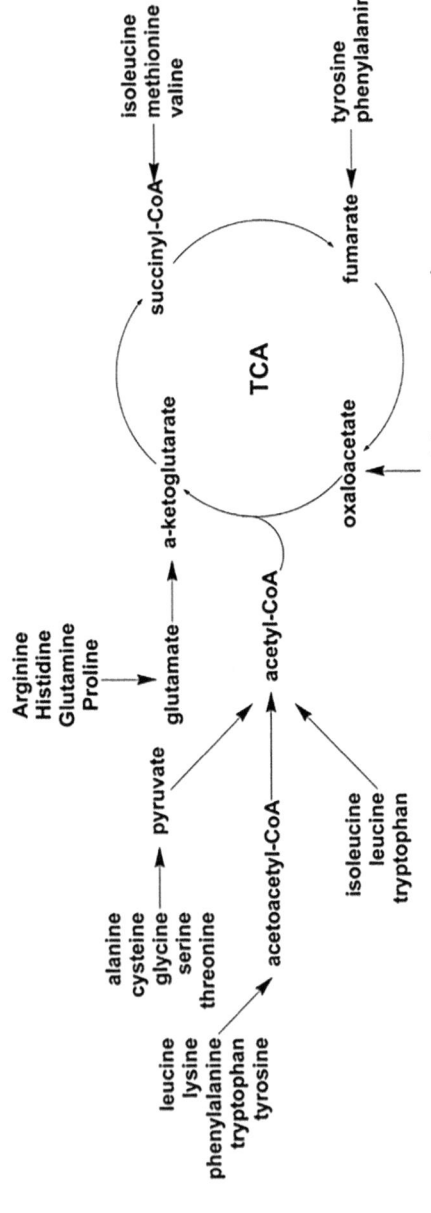

Fig. 3.17 The catabolism of amino acid skeletons. Once deaminated, the carbon backbones of amino acids are converted to acetyl-CoA or intermediates of the TCA

Cysteine is metabolized in a number of ways. One common excretory pathway involves the metabolism of cysteine to sulfite and pyruvate. Cysteine can also be dimerized through oxidation by **cystine reductase**. Cystine is just the disulfide bonded form of cysteine. **Cystinuria** is a defect in the renal proximal transporter for dibasic amino acids that leads to the urinary excretion of cystine, lysine, and arginine. Cystine is the least soluble and thus has a tendency to form **cystine kidney stones** in this disease, hence the name of the disease.

Methionine is metabolized to cysteine and succinyl-CoA, as shown in the cysteine synthesis pathway in Fig. 3.8. Defects in this pathway can lead to the homocysteinurias as discussed earlier.

Tyrosine is metabolized to fumarate, an intermediate in the TCA, an acetoacetyl-CoA, a ketone body. This process is shown in Fig. 3.18. Hence it is one of the amino acids that are both ketogenic and glucogenic. The thyroxine ring is broken down by an enzyme known as **homogentisate oxidase**, and mutations in this enzyme result in **Alkaptonuria (Ochronosis)**. This disease results from the accumulation of homogentisate, which causes **arthritis** and connective tissue discoloration. The urine also turns dark on exposure to air, and dark staining of diapers was frequently the presenting symptom until newborn screening began detecting the disease at birth. Other tyrosinemia syndromes result from defects in other enzymes within the pathway. Type I Tyrosinemia is a defect in fumarylacetoacetate hydrolase resulting in high levels of tyrosine in the blood, which can lead to **death from liver failure**. Treatment is a low tyrosine and phenylalanine diet. Type II tyrosinemia (Richner–Hanhart syndrome) is a defect in tyrosine aminotransferase. Neonatal tyrosinemia is a defect in p-hydroxyphenylpyruvate hydroxylase.

Phenylalanine is metabolized to tyrosine by **phenylalanine hydroxylase** as discussed earlier and shown in Fig. 3.9.

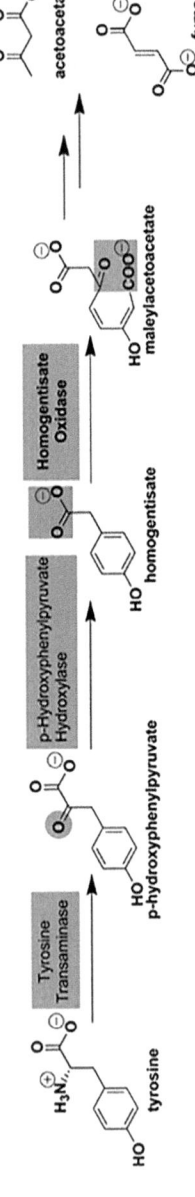

Fig. 3.18 Tyrosine is catabolized to fumarate and acetoacetate. Defects in homogentisate oxidase cause alkaptonuria (ochronosis)

Proline is catabolized in two steps through ring cleavage and oxidation to glutamate, which is then further catabolized to α-ketoglutarate. Mutations in either step can lead to severe disorders known collectively as the **hyperprolinemias**.

Branched-Chain Amino Acids: While the degradation of most amino acids primarily occurs in the liver, the degradation of branched-chain amino acids primarily occurs in muscle. The branched-chain α-keto acid dehydrogenase complex involved in branched-chain amino acid degradation is primarily expressed in muscle and sparsely in the liver. A schematic of branched-chain amino acid degradation is shown in Fig. 3.19. Successively, they are transaminated, decarboxylated and activated by coenzyme A, and finally dehydrogenated, to yield molecules that can be further metabolized. The glutamate generated through this process is cycled to the liver through the glutamate cycle discussed earlier to produce ammonia. **Maple**

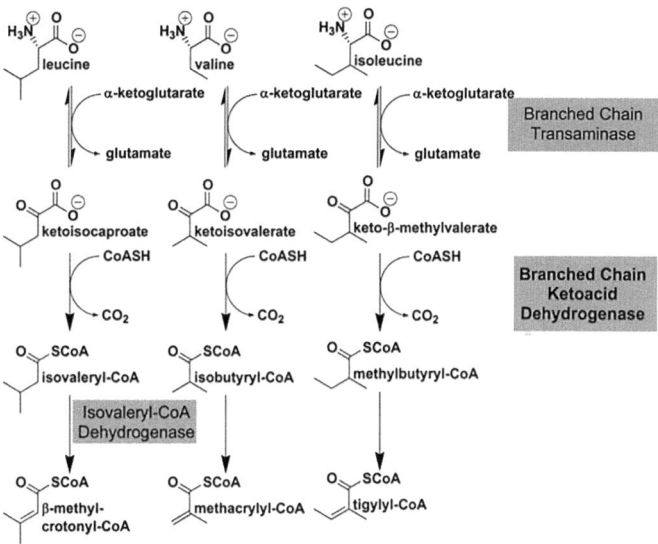

Fig. 3.19 Branched chain amino acid degradation. Defects in branched chain ketoacid dehydrogenase lead to maple syrup urine disease

Syrup Urine Disease is a defect in the **α-keto decarboxylase complex** that leads to brain damage and early mortality. Treatment must limit intake of leucine, isoleucine, and valine. **Mnemonic: I L**ove **V**ermont maple syrup—for the three amino acids that must be limited in the diet. **Intermittent Branched-Chain Ketonuria** is a mild defect in the α-keto decarboxylase complex that leads to milder symptoms than those seen in Maple Syrup Urine Disease. **Isovaleric Acidemia** is a defect in isovaleryl-CoA dehydrogenase (the final step in the metabolism of leucine) that leads to vomiting, acidosis, and coma with excess protein ingestion. Treatment is to limit leucine intake.

Insulin and Glucagon in Amino Acid Metabolism

Dietary amino acids stimulate the release of both insulin and glucagon from the pancreatic islets. In turn, insulin and glucagon are important regulators of amino acid uptake and metabolism by tissues, once again emphasizing the role of these hormones as pan-metabolic hormones. Insulin induces the uptake of amino acids by peripheral tissues such as muscle, where they are used for anabolism, while glucagon primarily stimulates the uptake of amino acids by the liver, where they are used for gluconeogenesis. In fasting states, glucagon signaling predominates, and glucagon induces release of amino acids from peripheral tissues such as muscle and their subsequent uptake by the liver for gluconeogenesis.

Porphyrin Synthesis and the Porphyrias

Heme is the central component of several proteins, including hemoglobin and myoglobin, and is central to their oxygen carrying capacity. Heme consists of a porphyrin ring and an atom of iron (Fe^{2+}), as shown in Fig. 3.20. Heme is synthesized from **gly-**

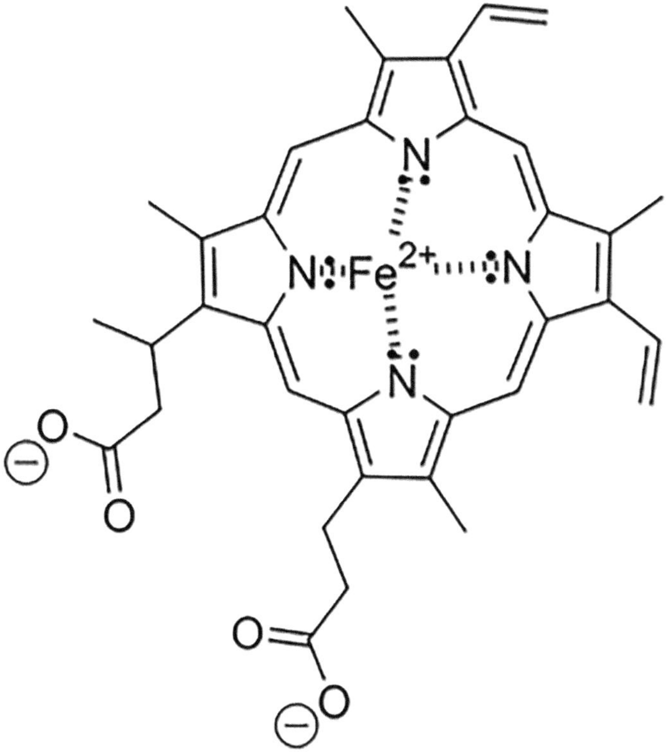

Fig. 3.20 Heme B, consisting of an iron atom within a porphyrin ring

cine and **succinyl Co-A**. Defects in the synthesis of heme lead to the porphyrias, which are characterized by **photosensitivity, painful abdomen, pink urine, polyneuropathy, psychological disturbances**, and **severe disfigurement**, and the physiological basis of these symptoms is schematized in Fig. 3.21. The specific nature of each porphyria is also given in Table 3.1. **You should be familiar with <u>porphyria cutanea tarda</u> and <u>acute intermittent porphyria</u>. Lead can inhibit <u>ferrochelatase</u> and <u>ALA dehydratase</u>**, thus leading to an acquired porphyria phenotype.

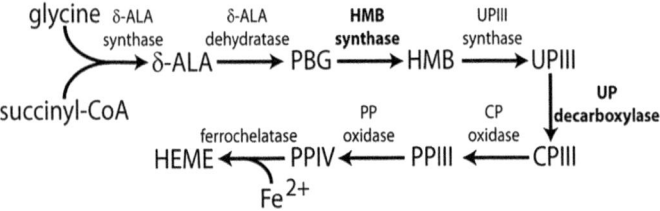

Fig. 3.21 Heme synthesis. Heme is synthesized in 8 steps from glycine and succinyl-CoA as shown above. Glycine and succinyl-CoA are first condensed by δ-ALA Synthase to form δ-ALA. δ-ALA is then converted to protobilinogen (PBG) by δ-ALA Dehydratase. PBG is then converted to hydroxymethylbilane (HMB) by HBM Synthase. HMB is then converted to uroporphyrinogen III (UPIII) by UPIII Synthase. UPIII in turn is converted to coproporphyrinogen III (CPIII) by UP decarboxylase. CPIII is converted to protoporphyrinogen III (PPIII) by CP oxidase, and PPIII is converted to PPIV by PP Oxidase. Finally, PPIV is chelated with iron by ferrochelatase to form heme

Table 3.1 The porphyrias

Disease	Inheritance	Deficiency	Symptoms
X-linked sideroblastic anemia	X-linked recessive	δ-ALA synthase	Sideroblastic anemia
δ-ALA dehydratase deficiency	AR	δ-ALA dehydratase	Abdominal pain
			Psychiatric symptoms
			lead also inhibits δ-ALA Dehydratase; lead poisoning presents with similar symptoms
Acute intermittent porphyria	AD	HMB synthase (PBG deaminase)	Abdominal pain
			Psychiatric symptoms
Congenital erythropoeitic porphyria	AR	Uroporphyrinogen III synthase (UPIII synthase)	Abdominal pain
			Peripheral neuropathy
			Psychiatric symptoms
			Tachycardia

Table 3.1 (continued)

Disease	Inheritance	Deficiency	Symptoms
Porphyria cutanea tarda	AD	Uroporphyrinogen decarboxylase (UP decarboxylase)	Photosensitivity
			Cutaneous vesicles, bullae
Heriditary coproporphyria	AD	Coproporphyrinogen oxidase (CP oxidase)	Photosensitivity
			Abdominal pain (colic)
Variegate porphyria	AD	Protoporphyrinogen oxidase (PP oxidase)	Photosensitivity
			Developmental delay
Erythropoeitic protoporphyria	AD	Ferrochelatase	Photosensitivity
			Cutaneous vesicles, bullae
			Gall stones, Liver dysfunction

*Metabolic diseases of porphyrin metabolism

Hemoglobin

Heme consists of a porphyrin ring chelated to an atom of ferrous iron (Fe^{2+}). This heme moiety is contained within the hemoglobin subunit. Four hemoglobin subunits (2α and 2β) comprise HbA (the adult hemoglobin). Fetal hemoglobin is comprised of 2α and 2γ subunits. Myoglobin is a monomeric protein that contains a single heme.

Methemoglobinemia results when the ferrous iron (Fe^{2+}) at the center of the heme moiety is oxidized to ferric iron (Fe^{3+}). Fe^{3+} is incapable of binding O_2, and hence the hemoglobin becomes dysfunctional. Within normal erythrocytes, **NADH-cytochrome b_5 reductase** normally reduces any Fe^{3+} back to Fe^{2+}, thus preventing the accumulation of ferric iron. **Congenital methemoglobinemia** can result from deficiencies in his enzyme. Acquired methemoglobinemia can occur with certain drugs, including nitrates, that oxidize iron. The characteristic symptom is **chocolate cyanosis**, in which the skin turns a brownish-blue color. Other symptoms include anxiety, headache, and shortness of breath (dyspnea). The treatment is the administration of **methylene blue**, which reduces Fe^{3+} back to Fe^{2+}.

Porphyrin Degradation

Erythrocytes are replaced approximately every 100–120 days. As part of this process, the hemoglobin must be degraded. **Macrophages of the reticuloendothelial system** catalyze the formation of **bilirubin** from the porphyrin ring. Specifically, (1) porphyrin is first converted to **biliverdin** by the **microsomal heme oxygenase system**. Then, (2) biliverdin is converted to **bilirubin** by **biliverdin reductase**. Bilirubin is then transported to the liver, where it is conjugated to **glucuronic acid** to increase its solubility and then excreted in **bile**. Defects in liver conjugation and excretion lead to a variety of diseases (**Crigler–Najjar Syndrome, Gilbert Syndrome, Dubin-Johnson Syndrome, Rotor Syndrome**, etc.) that are covered in detail in gastrointestinal pathophysiology courses.

Important Diseases of Amino Acid Metabolism

Major Metabolic Diseases

Hepatic Encephalopathy: Liver failure leads to toxins (ammonia) accumulation, brain dysfunction (encephalopathy) Kwashiorkor—a state of protein deficiency leading to edema, anemia, and steatosis (fatty liver).

Marasmus: A state of general caloric deficiency which leads to muscle wasting and edema.

Some Important Enzyme Deficiencies in Amino Acid Metabolism

Homocysteinuria: Deficiency in cystathionine b-synthase leads to accumulation of homocysteine.

Phenylketonuria: Deficiency in phenylalanine hydroxylase leads to accumulation of phenylalanine.

The Urea Cycle Defects

Alkaptonuria: Deficiency in homogentisate oxidase leads to the accumulation of homogentisate, a metabolite of tyrosine Maple Syrup Urine Disease—deficiency in the branched-chain keto acid dehydrogenase leads to the accumulation of toxic byproducts of branched-chain (valine, leucine, isoleucine) amino acid catabolism.

The Porphyrias

This is discussed in the section "Porphyrin Synthesis and the Porphyrias."

Nucleotide Metabolism

Biologically Important Nucleotides

A nucleotide has three components: a nitrogenous base, a pentose sugar, and a phosphate linkage. The nitrogenous bases include two categories: purines, which contain two aromatic rings, and pyrimidines, which have only one aromatic ring. The pentose sugars that are used biologically for nucleotide synthesis include ribose in RNA and deoxyribose in DNA, and these are shown in Fig. 4.1. Finally, phosphates are attached to the sugar. Phosphates may be attached to the free 2′, 3′, or 5′ positions of the sugar. Additionally, there may be multiple phosphates attached to the sugar, as in ATP, which has three phosphates linked in a chain to the 5′ position. Nucleosides are nucleotides without phosphates, essentially just the nitrogenous base and a pentose sugar.

The structures of the important nitrogenous bases, adenine (A), guanine (G), cytosine (C), uracil (U), and thymine (T) are shown in Fig. 4.1. Uracil is normally found only in ribonucleic acids, while thymine is only found in deoxyribonucleic acids. In nucleoside form, these are known as adenosine, guanosine, cytidine, uridine, and thymidine. **Ribonucleotides** contain ribose and are important in RNA synthesis (mRNA, rRNA, tRNA). In their triphosphate form, ribonucleotides also serve as high-energy donors (ATP, CTP, GTP, and UTP). All four nucleotide triphosphates serve as important high-energy donors in various reactions.

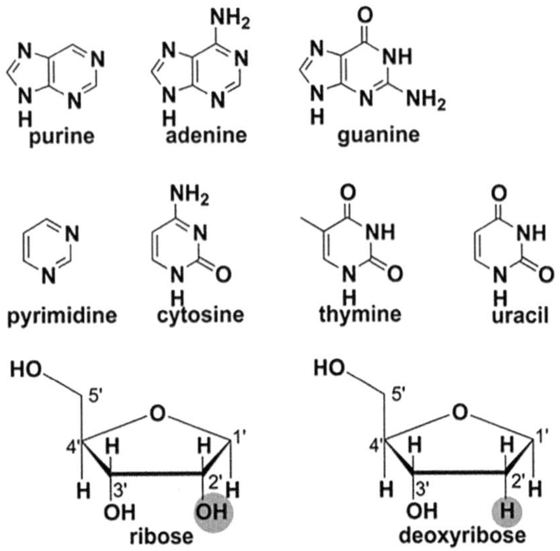

Fig. 4.1 The structures of the important nitrogenous bases and pentose sugars found in nucleotides

Ribonucleosides and ribonucleotides have many other biological functions as well. For example, adenosine, ADP, cyclic AMP (cAMP), and cyclic GMP (cGMP) are important signaling mediators, ATP is the precursor to the formation of the cofactors NADH, NADPH, and FAD, and all four nucleotides serve as substrates for phosphorylation reactions. **Deoxyribonucleotides** are primarily important in DNA synthesis and include dATP, dCTP, dGTP, and dTTP.

Nucleotides may be linked in polymers. **Phosphodiester bonds** connect one pentose to another pentose. As part of the DNA or RNA backbone, phosphates are linked in 3′–5′ phosphodiester bonds. There are other phosphodiester linkages as well. For example, in the mRNA cap, there is a 5′–5′ phosphate linkage, and in some catalytic RNAs, there is a 2′–5′ linkage. **Glycosidic bonds** connect a pentose to a nitrogenous base and nitrogenous bases are generally attached at the 1′ carbon.

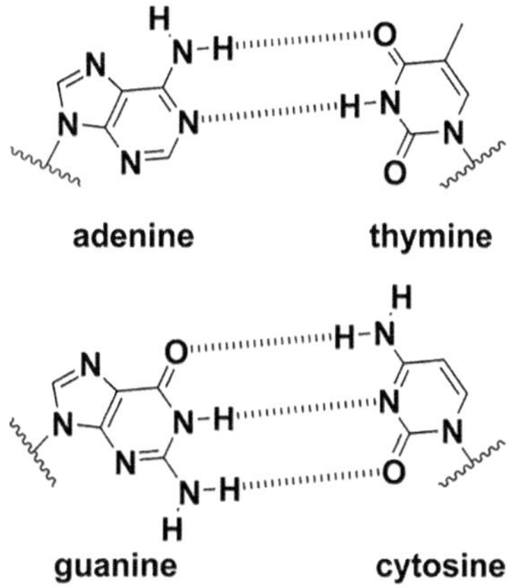

Fig. 4.2 Watson-Crick base pairing

adenine　　　thymine

guanine　　　cytosine

Bases are capable of hydrogen bonding, an important property in the function of both DNA and RNA. Adenine forms two hydrogen bonds to uracil and thymine, while guanine forms three hydrogen bonds to cytosine, as shown in Fig. 4.2. The hydrogen bonding patterns create grooves in the macromolecule DNA. The major groove and the minor groove are defined based on the separation of the ribose rings on the base pairs. The major groove is a common place to find proteins bound, whereas the minor groove is bound more commonly by small molecules. There are also non-Watson-Crick base pairs allowed, and they are important in the structure of many nucleic acid macromolecules.

Purine Nucleotide Biosynthesis

All purines can be biosynthesized. Purines are synthesized de novo primarily in rapidly dividing cells as in hematopoietic cells and in tumors and to some degree in hepatocytes. Quiescent cells typically reuse purines through a process known as salvage, which will be discussed later. *This difference is essential to understand and remember—cancer chemotherapeutics can inhibit de novo purine synthesis and ultimately DNA synthesis and thus selec-*

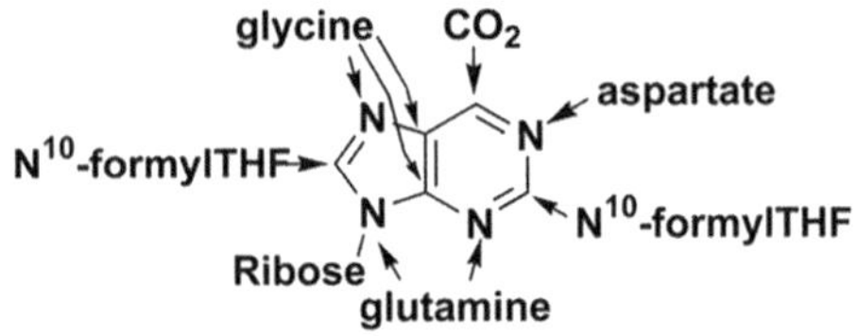

Fig. 4.3 Derivation of the purine base

tively target tumor cells while leaving most normal tissues untouched. However, cells of the immune system are highly affected, which is why immunosuppression is a common side effect of many cancer chemotherapeutics.

The derivative of each carbon and nitrogen in a purine base in de novo biosynthesis is schematized in Fig. 4.3. The synthesis, diagrammed in Figs. 4.4 and 4.5, is complex and certainly not one you should bother memorizing unless this field particularly interests you. There are some key steps with which you should be familiar. The purine rings can be synthesized from scratch. The starting material is **ribose-5'-monophosphate**. This is first converted to **inosine monophosphate**, which is then converted either to **guanosine monophosphate** or **adenosine monophosphate**. The synthesis of inosine monophosphate is diagrammed in Fig. 4.4, while the remaining synthesis to GMP and AMP is outlined in Fig. 4.5.

The first step is the activation of ribose monophosphate through pyrophosphorylation to produce phosphoribosyl pyrophosphate (PRPP), which is catalyzed by **PRPP synthase**. This is a highly regulated step of purine biosynthesis and again follows the basic principles of substrate activation and product inhibition. **ATP** and **GTP** are the major inhibitors of this enzyme, while **phosphate** is the major activator. PRPP is a common precursor to both purine and pyrimidine nucleotides.

The second step is the conversion of this activated phosphoribosyl pyrophosphate to **phosphoribosylamine** by transferring an amine from **glutamine**, which is in turn converted to glutamate. This step is catalyzed by **PRPP glutamyl amidotransferase**. This reaction is somewhere between a true S_N1 and a true S_N2

Purine Nucleotide Biosynthesis

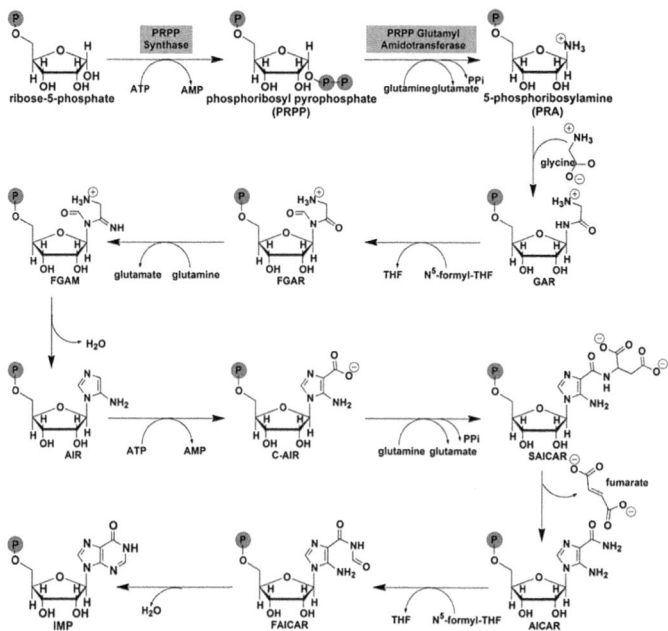

Fig. 4.4 Synthesis of inosine monophosphate (IMP), the common precursor for both AMP and GMP, from Ribose-5′-phosphate

reaction, but more importantly, this is the **rate determining step** and **first committed step** of purine biosynthesis. This second step, as the rate determining step, is also highly regulated, being feedback inhibited by IMP, GMP, and AMP.

After this, phosphoribosylamine is converted to inosine monophosphate (IMP), the common precursor for both AMP and GMP synthesis. This is a complex process that requires ATP and tetrahydrofolate (THF).

Inosine monophosphate (IMP) is then converted to either AMP or GMP. **Notice here that GTP is required for AMP synthesis, while ATP is required for GMP synthesis.** Thus, guanine nucleotides are selectively synthesized when ATP stores are high, while adenosine nucleotides are selectively synthesized when GTP stores are high.

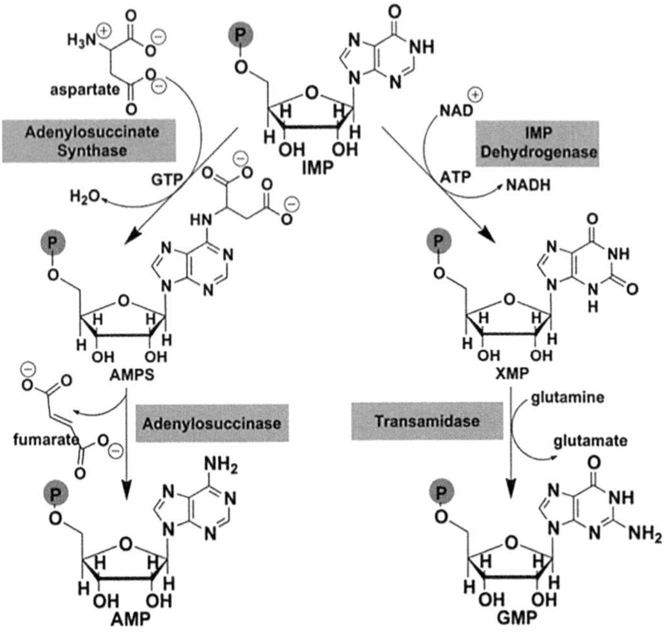

Fig. 4.5 Synthesis of AMP and GMP from IMP

Regulation of De Novo Purine Biosynthesis

As you can see, de novo synthesis is an extensive and energy consuming process. Thus, it is highly regulated teleologically to prevent the unnecessary use of energy in this process. PRPP synthase and PRPP glutamyl amidotransferase are highly regulated as discussed above. Specifically, PRPP synthase is inhibited by ATP and GTP, while PRPP glutamyl amidotransferase is inhibited by AMP, GMP, and IMP. In addition, AMP and GMP inhibit every step of the pathway. The balance between ATP and GTP is also highly regulated. GTP is necessary for ATP synthesis, while ATP is necessary for GTP synthesis. ATP and GTP also inhibit their own synthesis.

Chemotherapeutic Agents that Block Purine Synthesis Enzymes

Because most normal tissues rely almost exclusively on nucleotide salvage pathways, many cancer chemotherapeutics inhibit de novo purine synthesis (and pyrimidine synthesis) and ultimately DNA synthesis and thus selectively target tumor cells while leaving most normal tissues untouched (the immune system is the notable exception and is heavily affected by many chemotherapies).

1. **Mycophenolic acid** (usually used as mycophenolate mofetil) inhibits **IMP dehydrogenase.**
2. **6-mercaptopurine** inhibits **IMP dehydrogenase** and **PRPP glutamyl amidotransferase**
3. **Methotrexate**, a commonly used chemotherapy agent, blocks **dihydrofolate reductase**, the enzyme which converts dihydrofolate to tetrahydrofolate. Notice that **folic acid** is an essential cofactor for the function of **formyl transferase**, and this is a key step in nucleotide synthesis that is thus blocked when tetrahydrofolate levels are reduced by methotrexate. **Methotrexate blocks both purine and pyrimidine biosynthesis.**

Purine Salvage

In addition to de novo biosynthesis of purines, purine nucleotides can also be synthesized from preformed purines, adenine, guanine, and hypoxanthine. We obtain large amounts of DNA and RNA in our diet, and this is a mechanism by which nucleotides in the diet can be salvaged and utilized for anabolic processes. DNA and RNA in our diet are first broken down by pancreatic enzymes and enterocyte enzymes to pentose sugars and nitrogenous bases. From there, the bases can be salvaged to make new nucleotides simply by forming new glycosidic bonds.

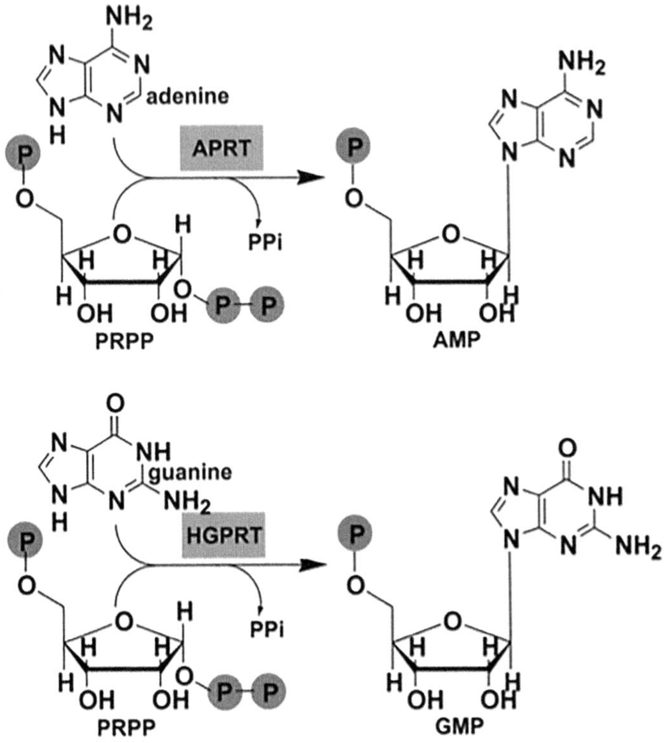

Fig. 4.6 Purine salvage

Adenine phosphoribosyltransferase (APRT) catalyzes the addition of adenine to **PRPP** to form AMP, as shown in Fig. 4.6.

Hypoxanthine-guanine phosphoribosyltransferase (HGPRT) catalyzes the addition of guanine to PRPP to form GMP or hypoxanthine to PRPP to form IMP, as shown in Fig. 4.6. Deficiency in **HGPRT** causes **Lesch–Nyhan syndrome 1**, an X-linked disorder. This leads to the inability to salvage guanine nucleotides and inosine nucleotides, leading to the accumulation of guanine and hypoxanthine, which enter the purine degradation pathway. This leads to the excessive formation of **uric acid (urate)**, the product of purine degradation, which can accumulate in joints and tissues to cause gout (discussed subsequently) and also precipitate in the urine to cause kidney stones. Symptoms of the disease include **motor dysfunction**, **cognitive deficits**, and <u>*most strikingly, behavioral disturbances, such as self-mutilation (biting of the lips, fingers, arms, etc.).*</u>

Synthesis of Deoxyribonucleotides

Deoxyribonucleotides are formed from ribonucleotides by the enzyme **ribonucleotide reductase**, as shown in Fig. 4.7. This enzyme requires **thioredoxin**, a sulfoprotein that can participate in redox reactions much the same way that NADH, NADPH, and FAD do. This enzyme is also feedback inhibited by **dATP** and is highly regulated. Ribonucleotide reductase activity is generally only upregulated during the S phase of mitosis to increase the dNTP pool as needed. Importantly, this enzyme is also inhibited by hydroxyurea, which inactivates the active site tyrosine free radical. Hydroxyurea thus inhibits DNA synthesis in the rapidly dividing tumor cells and is used as a chemotherapeutic agent in certain cancers.

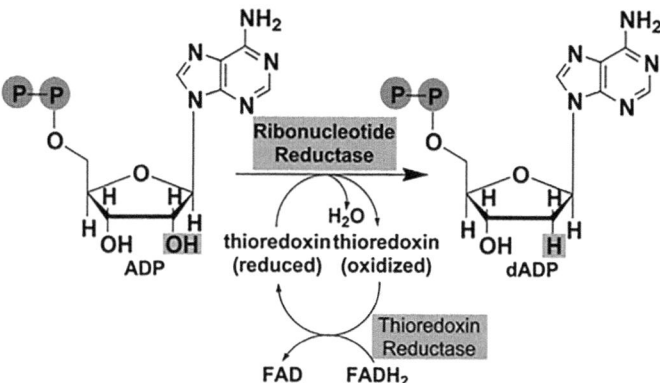

Fig. 4.7 Synthesis of deoxyribonucleotides

Purine Degradation: The Production of Uric Acid

The essence of purine degradation is simple and is diagrammed in Fig. 4.8. The liver is essentially the only organ in the body that carries out purine degradation.

1. AMP and GMP are dephosphorylated to yield the free nucleosides, adenosine and guanosine.
2. Adenosine is then deaminated to yield inosine by **Adenosine Deaminase**.
3. Subsequently, inosine and guanosine are deribosylated, yielding the free bases hypoxanthine and guanine, respectively, and free ribose-1-phosphate.
4. Hypoxanthine is converted to xanthine by **Xanthine Oxidase**.
5. Guanine is deaminated to xanthine.
6. Xanthine is converted to **Uric Acid (urate)** by **Xanthine Oxidase.**

Adenosine Deaminase Deficiency leads to **Severe Combined Immunodeficiency (SCID)** because excess accumulation of ATP inhibits guanine nucleotide synthesis and salvage pathways and also inhibits ribonucleotide reductase. This prevents DNA synthesis, leading to generalized deficiency in all immune cells. Immune cells are particularly affected because they are among the most rapidly dividing cells within the body. *Of note, this is the first disease that was treated by experimental gene therapy.*

Uric acid is relatively water insoluble. Uric acid is eventually eliminated both in the urine (65%) and in the bile (35%). Normal urate levels in the blood are 4–6 mg/dL. Hyperuricemia is diagnosed when urate levels are >7 mg/dL for men and >6 mg/dL for women.

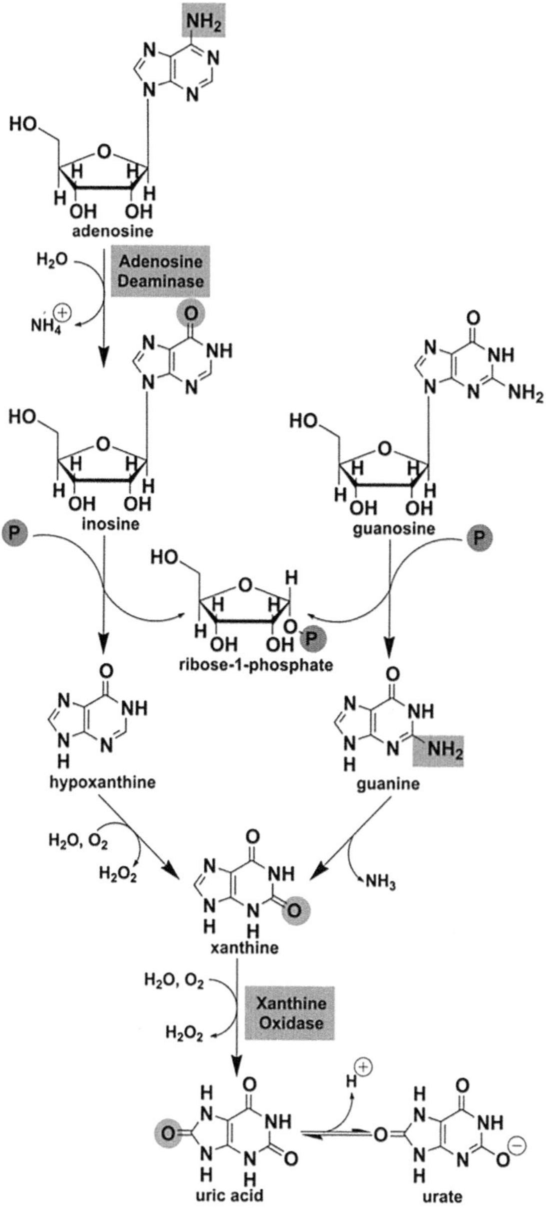

Purine Degradation: The Production of Uric Acid

Fig. 4.8 Purine nucleotide catabolism to uric acid

Urate Pools

There are several sources of nucleotides and/or uric acid that eventually can give rise to uric acid through purine degradation. These pools include de novo synthesis, diet, purine salvage, and urinary reabsorption. All of these are potentially targetable in the context of gout, the accumulation of excess uric acid in the body, as shown below:

De novo synthesis—xanthine oxidase inhibitors
Dietary purines—low-purine or low alcohol diet
Salvage—gene therapy for HGPRT (?)
Urinary reabsorption—inhibit renal transporters

Causes of Hyperuricemia

Inborn Errors of Metabolism 1: Disorders of purine metabolism like hypoxanthine-guanine phosphoribosyltransferase (HGPRT) deficiency (**Lesch–Nyhan Syndrome**) and phosphoribosyl pyrophosphate (PPRP) synthetase overactivity are known inborn errors of metabolism which lead to hyperuricemia and are known to be genetic causes of gout in humans.

Dietary Causes of Hyperuricemia: The excess uric acid can be due to an increase in consumption of foods that are high in purines (meats, seafoods, beans, etc.). Alcohol use can also increase uric acid levels (both by causing overproduction and underexcretion of uric acid) and increase the chance of a gout attack.

Excretory Causes of Hyperuricemia: Reduced renal excretion due to renal failure can be a major cause of hyperuricemia.

Pathophysiology and Clinical Manifestations of Gout

Gout is caused by a buildup of uric acid in the body (hyperuricemia). The high levels of uric acid, over time, lead to deposits in joints and can form needle-like crystals. As these crystals accumulate in joint capsules, they actually activate complement. This leads to phagocytosis of the crystals by macrophages, but perhaps more importantly, the recruitment of neutrophils to the synovium. The neutrophils in turn release a variety of inflammatory factors that create pain and also tissue and cartilage destruction. Other sites of uric acid accumulation include in the skin (tophi, classically found on the big toe or ear) or in the kidney as kidney stones.

Gout is usually divided into four phases:

1. Asymptomatic hyperuricemia.
2. Acute gouty attack due to accumulation of sufficient crystals in the joints (these resolve spontaneously over hours to days for unknown reasons). 50% of patients find this occurring first in the big toe (first metatarsophalangeal joint).
3. Intercritical period between attacks.
4. Chronic gout due to destruction of the joint and chronic inflammatory processes.

Treatment

Lifestyle Management: Dietary restrictions on high-purine foods (eggs, dairy and potatoes are low-purine foods), avoiding/limiting alcohol intake, maintaining hydration and regular food intake.

Acute Gout: Treating the gouty attacks once they have occurred largely centers around reducing the painful inflammatory processes. 1. **NSAIDs** acutely reduce pain and inflammation in the joint by inhibiting the cyclooxygenase pathways and thus prostaglandin synthesis.

2. **Colchicine** <u>binds to tubulin and blocks microtubule mediated cell motility</u> (such as neutrophil diapedesis) and cell division

(both processes require depolymerization and repolymerization of microtubules). This will thus reduce the inflammatory response by limiting the ability of immune cells, such as neutrophils, from infiltrating into the synovium.
3. **Glucocorticoids** potently inhibit phospholipase A_2 through the generation of lipocortins, thus blocking the production of eicosanoids and reducing pain and inflammation.

Chronic Gout: Treating chronic gout centers largely around reducing the production of uric acid by targeting the purine synthesis, salvage, and degradative pathways.

1. **Probenecid** inhibits urate reabsorption in the proximal tubules of the kidney and increases secretion of urate. Probenecid may predispose to the formation of uric acid kidney stones.
2. **Allopurinol** is an analog of xanthine. Allopurinol is oxidized by **xanthine oxidase** to oxypurinol (alloxanthine), which then efficiently inhibits the same enzyme, **xanthine oxidase**. This results in the accumulation of hypoxanthine in the blood. Because hypoxanthine is much more water soluble than uric acid, it is readily excreted and high levels are not dangerous.
3. **Uricase**: Non-human mammals have uricase, which breaks down urate and prevents gout. **Rasburicase**, a recombinant Aspergillus uricase, is now approved in the USA. This can be used to prevent gout by degrading uric acid to **allantoin**, a water soluble compound that is freely excreted in the urine.

Pyrimidine Biosynthesis

Unlike purine biosynthesis, in which the purine ring is synthesized on the ribose, pyrimidine rings are synthesized and then ribosylated. The derivation of the atoms of the pyrimidine is schematized in Fig. 4.9 and pyrimidine synthesis itself is shown in Fig. 4.10.

The first step in pyrimidine biosynthesis is the formation of **carbamoyl phosphate**. Sound familiar? Yes—this is the same reaction as the first step in the urea cycle. However, this is catalyzed by **Carbamoyl Phosphate Synthase II (CPSII)**. **CPSI** (the enzyme in the urea cycle) is located in the mitochondria, while

Fig. 4.9 Derivation of the pyrimidine base

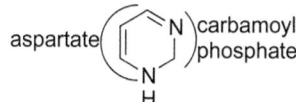

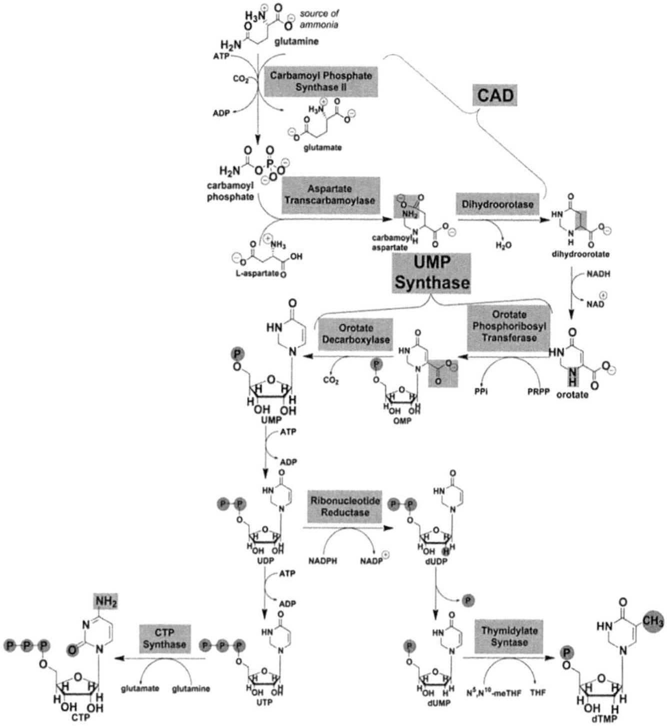

Fig. 4.10 Pyrimidine nucleotide biosynthesis. UDP is synthesized from carbamoyl phosphate and serves as the common precursor for both cytidine and thymidine nucleotides. UDP is then converted in two steps to either CTP or dTMP as shown above

CPSII (the enzyme involved in pyrimidine biosynthesis) is located in the cytosol. *Thus, carbamoyl phosphate synthesis occurs both in the mitochondria and in the cytosol by separate enzymes and for use in different processes!* CPSII is not regulated by N-acetylglutamate like CPSI is.

Carbamoyl phosphate is then converted to carbamoyl aspartate by aspartate transcarbamoylase, and carbamoyl aspartate is converted to dihydroorotate by dihydroorotase. These three enzymes, CPSII, aspartate transcarbamoylase, and dihydroorotase are all domains of a single protein, known as CAD for the first letters of each enzymatic domain. Dihydroorotate is then converted to orotate, the common precursor for all of the pyrimidines.

Uridine monophosphate (UMP) synthase then converts orotate to UMP. UMP synthase is a bifunctional enzyme that contains within it two subenzymes, orotate phosphoribosyltransferase and orotidylic acid decarboxylase. Mutations in UMP synthase result in **orotic aciduria**, the main symptoms (including poor growth and megaloblastic anemia) of which result from the inability to produce pyrimidine nucleotides.

UMP is then converted to CTP and TMP. Importantly, the synthesis of TMP requires **tetrahydrofolate** and is catalyzed by **thymidylate synthase**.

Regulation of Pyrimidine Biosynthesis

Pyrimidine synthesis is regulated at the level of CPSII. UTP is a competitive inhibitor of CPSII by binding in the ATP binding site but failing to act as a phosphate donor. PRPP, however, activates CPSII, showing us once again the concept of product inhibition and substrate activation. Pyrimidine salvage occurs in two steps, as shown in Fig. 4.11. First, pyrimidine bases are combined with ribose-1-phosphate by **nucleoside phosphorylase** to form a pyrimidine nucleoside. These nucleosides are then phosphorylated at the 5′ position by **nucleoside kinase** to yield pyrimidine nucleotides. Notice that this is very different from the purine salvage pathway discussed earlier, which occurs in a single step and relies on PRPP as a starting material rather than ribose-1-phosphate.

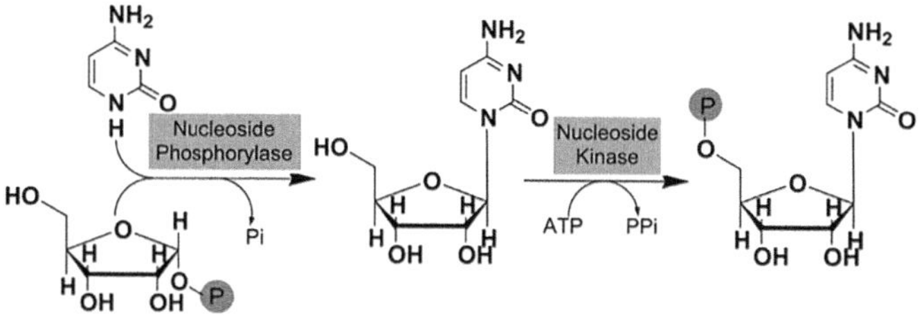

Fig. 4.11 Pyrimidine salvage occurs in two distinct steps, in contrast to purine salvage

Chemotherapeutic Agents that Block Pyrimidine Synthesis Enzymes

1. **5-fluorouracil (5-FU)** inhibits **thymidylate synthase**, thus blocking dUMP to TMP conversion. Specifically, 5-FU is first converted to 5-FUTP and then converted to 5-FdUTP, which then binds to the thymidylate synthase active site.
2. **Leflunomide** inhibits **dihydroorotate dehydrogenase**, thus preventing the formation of orotic acid.
3. **Methotrexate**, discussed earlier as a purine synthesis inhibitors, blocks **dihydrofolate reductase. Methotrexate blocks both purine and pyrimidine biosynthesis**.

Pyrimidine Salvage

Just like purines can be salvaged, so can pyrimidines. The same dichotomy between de novo synthesis and salvage that applies to purines also applies to pyrimidines—namely that most mature tissues rely on salvage, while rapidly growing cells rely on both salvage and de novo synthesis. Pyrimidine salvage occurs in two steps as shown for cytosine in Fig. 4.11. Notice that this is unlike purine salvage, which only occurs in one step as shown in Fig. 4.6.

The pyrimidine base is first combined with ribose-1-phosphate by **nucleoside phosphorylase** to form the pyrimidine nucleoside.

The pyrimidine nucleoside is then phosphorylated at the 5′ position by **nucleoside kinase** to yield the nucleotide. Notice the differences here between purine and pyrimidine salvage.

Pyrimidine Degradation

Pyrimidines are degraded to water soluble products that are ultimately excreted in the urine through breaking of the ring structures. Uracil and cytosine are converted to β-alanine, while thymine is converted to β-aminoisobutyrate. **β-aminoisobutyrate is then converted to succinyl-CoA, which then enters the TCA! Thus, thymine can be catabolized and can enter the TCA!**

Rational Drug Design

Because so many drugs were discussed in this chapter and nucleotide biochemistry continues to be an active area of pharmacological and pharmaceutical investigation, especially within the context of cancer chemotherapeutics, it is useful to discuss the phases of clinical drug trials here. After a drug has been extensively tested in animal models, human clinical trials are carried out in four phases.

1. Phase 1 trials: in normal subjects or patients ($n = 20-80$)
   (a) Toxicity, with dose escalation
   (b) Metabolic, pharmacokinetics, pharmacologic action of drug in patients
2. Phase 2 trials: in patients, small scale (n = several hundred)
   (a) Preliminary efficacy and some further toxicity
3. Phase 3 trials: in patients, large scale (n = several hundred to several thousand)
   (a) Compare the drug to the best current regimen
   (b) Get accurate dosage and efficacy
4. Phase 4 trials:
   (a) After a drug is being used by patients, look at long-term benefits/risks.

Important Diseases of Nucleotide Metabolism

Major Metabolic Diseases

Gout: Accumulation of insoluble uric acid from a variety of causes leads to the precipitation of crystals in joints, leading to inflammation and destruction of the joint, and precipitation of crystals in the kidney, causing kidney stone formation.

Some Important Enzyme Deficiencies in Carbohydrate Metabolism

Lesch–Nyhan Syndrome: Deficiency in HGPRT leads to hyperuricemia, neurological disturbances, and self-mutilation. Severe combined immunodeficiency (SCID)—deficiency in adenosine deaminase (ADA) leads to immunosuppression because adenosine accumulates and inhibits the de novo synthesis of other nucleotides.

Vitamins 5

The material in this chapter is largely accessory material meant to add to your understanding and hence classified as an appendix. The details of vitamins and their associated deficiency and excess states are very important for the boards and are tested. These are presented in Tables 5.1 and 5.2. The remaining material reviews the chemistry of NADH, $FADH_2$, pyridoxal phosphate (PLP), and folic acid, is for your further edification.

Table 5.1 The fat soluble vitamins

Vitamin	Active form	Function	Deficiency	Excess
A (retinol)	Retinoic acid	Visual pigments (rhodopsin in retinal rods)	Night blindness	Alopecia (hair loss)
		Epithelial maintenance	Xeropthalmia (dry eyes)	Headache
			Impotence	Dry, pruritic skin
D	Calcitriol	Calcium and phosphate uptake (discussed in Chap. 2)	Rickets (kids)	Hypercalcemia
			Osteomalacia (adults)	Stupor
E		Antioxidant	Hemolysis (RBC membranes get oxidized and damaged)	Abdominal cramps hemorrhagic stroke
K		γ-carboxylation of clotting factors (factors II, VII, IX, X, C, and S)	Bleeding, hemorrhage (common in newborns)	Newborn jaundice hemolytic anemia

Table 5.2 The water soluble vitamins

Vitamin	Active form	Function	Deficiency	Excess
B1 thiamine	TPP	Enzymatic cofactor	BeriBeri (tachycardia, vomiting, convulsions)	Tachycardia, hypotension, headache, convulsions (extremely rare except with vitamin enthusiasts who overdose on multivitamins)
			Wernicke-Korsakoff syndrome (ataxia, confusion, ophthalmoplegia, amnestic confabulatory psychosis)	
B2 riboflavin	−FAD	Redox cofactor	Weakness, fatigue	Generally non-toxic
	−FMN		Dermatitis	
			Angular stomatitis	
B3 Niacin	−NAD$^+$	Redox cofactor	pellagra (dermatitis, diarrhea, dementia)	Flushing, pruritus, wheezing
	−NADP$^+$			Liver toxicity (jaundice)
B5 pantothenate	Coenzyme A	Acyl transfer cofactor	Dermatitis, enteritis, alopecia	Generally non-toxic
B6 pyridoxine	Pyridoxal phosphate (PLP)	Enzyme cofactor (transamination reactions)	convulsions, neuropathy	Sensory neuropathy (burning pain, numbness)
			Note that deficiency can be induced by INH, OCPs	Tachypnea

(continued)

Table 5.2 (continued)

Vitamin	Active form	Function	Deficiency	Excess
B12 cobalamin		Enzymatic cofactor	Megaloblastic anemia	*Generally non-toxic*
			Dementia	
			Spinal cord degeneration	
			Note that only animal sources have B12—vegetarians are at risk for developing deficiency	
C ascorbic acid		Cofactor for hydroxylation in collagen synthesis	Scurvy	Nephrolithiasis (kidney stones)
				Diarrhea, nausea
Folic acid	Tetrahydro-folate	Cofactor for one carbon transfers (purine, thymidine, methionine synthesis)	Megaloblastic anemia neural tube defects	*Generally non-toxic, but can mask B12 deficiency by hiding B12 deficiency associated megaloblastic anemia*

NAD⁺/NADH and FAD/FADH₂: The Biological REDOX Reagents

A Quick Review of REDOX Chemistry

Reduction–oxidation, or Redox, reactions involve the transfer of electrons between two compounds. One compound **gains electrons** and becomes **reduced**. The other compound **loses the same number of electrons** and becomes **oxidized**. The compound that is reduced oxidizes the other compound and is thus the **oxidizing agent**, while the compound that is oxidized reduces the other and is thus the **reducing agent**. A reduction is always coupled to an oxidation and vice versa because there can be no gain or loss of electrons from the system. However, each can be separated into a **half-reaction**: the **reduction half-reaction** and the **oxidation half-reaction**. Half reactions are always written by convention in the reduction pathway as shown below and are given a reduction potential, E°. The more positive the E°, the more spontaneously will a compound get reduced. Below, you see that oxygen has a very positive E° and thus readily gets reduced. Thus, oxygen is a strong oxidizing agent!

$$NAD^+ + H^+ + 2e^- \rightarrow NADH \rightarrow E° = -0.32\,V$$

$$FAD + 2H^+ + 2e^- \rightarrow FADH_2 \rightarrow E° = -0.18\,V$$

$$O_2 + 4H^+ + 4e^- \rightarrow 4H_2O \rightarrow E° = +0.82\,V$$

The E° means very little in and of itself because reductions must be coupled to oxidations in order to occur! Let us examine the coupling between the reduction of molecular oxygen and the oxidation of NADH below. Recall that we must reverse the sign of the reduction potential if we examine an oxidation. Also recall that we do not multiply the potential as we multiply a half-reaction. The absolute value of the potential always remains the same:

$$O_2 + 4H^+ + 4e^- \rightarrow 4H_2O \rightarrow E° = +0.82\,V$$

$$2NADH+ \rightarrow 2NAD^+ + 2H^+ + 4e^- \rightarrow E° = +0.32\,V$$

$$O_2 + 2H^+ + 2NADH \rightarrow 4H_2O + 2NAD^+ \rightarrow E° = +1.14\,V$$

This is highly exothermic! Remember the equation that relates free-energy ($\otimes G$) changes with the overall potential of a redox reaction: $\otimes G = -nFE°$. Thus, a large positive $E°$ means a large negative $\otimes G$. Because entropy does not play a large role in redox chemistry, this means that this is a large negative change in enthalpy—meaning a large amount of released energy! This is why the electron transport chain proceeds in the forward direction! It is highly favorable to transfer electrons from NADH (and FADH$_2$) to oxygen!

Coupling Redox Reactions: The Importance of Energetic Matching

Coupling of multiple **matched redox reactions** rather than a single mismatched redox reaction allows for the maximization of efficiency in energy usage. The closer the potentials between two reactions, the less energy is released as heat and thus lost to the surroundings. This is very important to a cell which is operating under strict energetic considerations. For this same reason, the electron transport chain in mitochondria involves multiple steps that slowly extract energy from the electron as it moves down its **potential gradient**. Ultimately, the net reaction of ATP generation is the burning of glucose with molecular oxygen, releasing CO_2 and H_2O. This is because oxygen has such a large oxidizing potential. However, doing this in one step releases large amounts of unharnessable energy; doing it in multiple smaller energetically matched steps allows for efficient capture of energy. For this reason, coupling of NAD$^+$ and FAD is important.

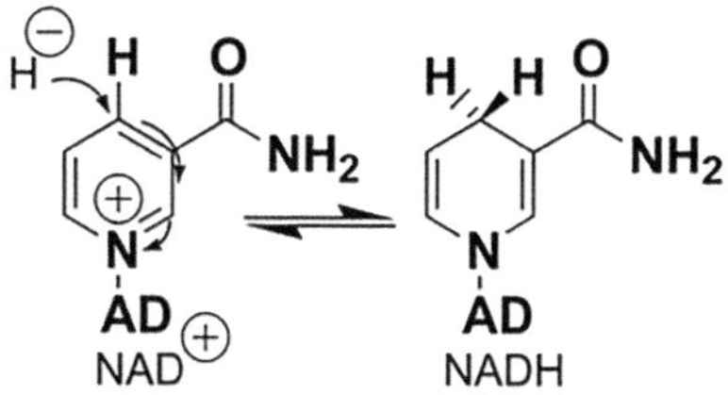

Fig. 5.1 NAD$^+$ and NADH

NAD$^+$/NADH

The chemistry of nicotinamide adenine dinucleotide (NAD) is simple. It has a pyridine ring, shown in Fig. 5.1, which can act as an electron sink and source. In NAD$^+$, this N is positively charged and primed to accept electron density. It is an electron withdrawing group that places a slight positive charge on the ortho-para positions. It is this positive charge at the para position which enables NAD$^+$ to readily accept a hydride to become NADH. Similarly NADH can release a hydride to become NAD$^+$. These are **redox** reactions, and for this reason the oxidation potential of NAD$^+$ or the reduction potential of NADH must closely match that of the coupled reaction to (1) ensure spontaneity of the reaction ($\mathbf{E°>0}$) and (2) ensure minimal energy loss by coupling reactions with similar energetics ($\mathbf{E°}$ **should be small**).

FAD/FADH$_2$ Reductions

FAD has a slightly different mode of operation than NAD$^+$—it is also a two electron acceptor, but it accepts along with the two electrons, two protons. Generally, a hydride source will add directly to the nitrogen in a **conjugate addition**, which allows the other nitrogen to pick up a proton from solution as shown in Fig. 5.2. FADH$_2$ can also participate in oxygen coupling reactions, which are not discussed here.

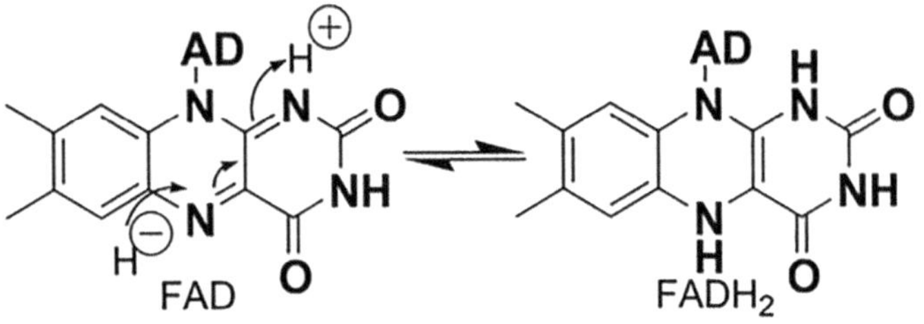

Fig. 5.2 FAD and FADH$_2$

Pyridoxine, Pyridoxal, and Pyridoxamine: The Chemistry of Vitamin B$_6$

Vitamin B$_6$ is ingested as pyridoxine and is subsequently oxidized enzymatically to pyridoxal, which is further phosphorylated by pyridoxal kinase, yielding the biologically active form, pyridoxal phosphate (PLP). Subsequent reductive amination of the cofactor results in another biological active form, pyridoxamine phosphate (PAP). These are shown in Fig. 5.3.

PLP is a versatile biological coenzyme involved in numerous amino acid based transformations including decarboxylations, side-chain elimination, ®-position and ©-position eliminations, oxidative deaminations, and reductive aminations (PAP), among others. PLP chemistry is the chemistry of the aldehyde (imine formation, imine hydrolysis, enolization, etc.) and of the pyridine ring, to which it owes its unique properties as an "electron sink." Fortunately, all mechanisms of PLP depend on this property and share a common initiation, the formation of a negative charge at the < position, which is subsequently resolved through various means.

Pyridoxal Phosphate (PLP): Chemical Reactivity

PLP utilizing enzymes almost always have a lysine residue present in the active site that condenses with the PLP to form an imine

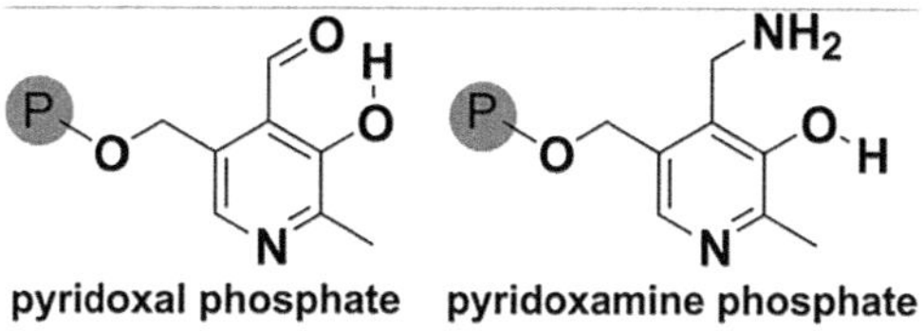

Fig. 5.3 Pyridoxal phosphate and pyridoxamine phosphate

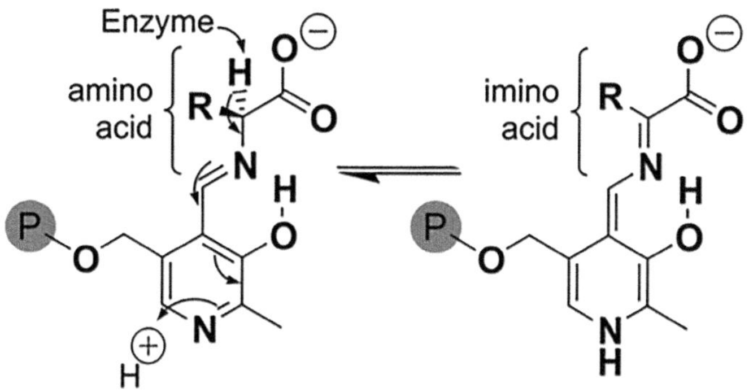

Fig. 5.4 PLP's stabilizes a negative charge at the α position of amino acids and thus catalyzes transaminations

(Schiff Base) covalent enzyme–co-enzyme linkage. Subsequently, the pyridoxamine (the imine of pyridoxal) will condense with the free amino group of an amino acid to carry out its catalysis of various reactions. The structure of PLP condensed with an amino acid is shown in Fig. 5.4.

The Reactions: There are many different classes of reactions catalyzed by PLP, but they all fall nicely into a few simple generalizable mechanisms

< position reactions: Stabilization of a negative charge at the < position. PLP will stabilize a negative charge at the < position of an amino acid, as shown in Fig. 5.5.

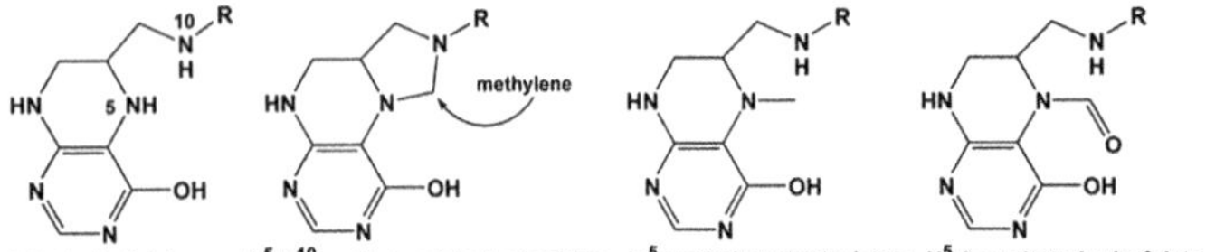

tetrahydrofolate N^5,N^{10}-methylenetetrahydrofolate N^5-methyltetrahydrofolate N^5-formyltetrahydrofolate

Fig. 5.5 Biologically important derivatives of folic acid

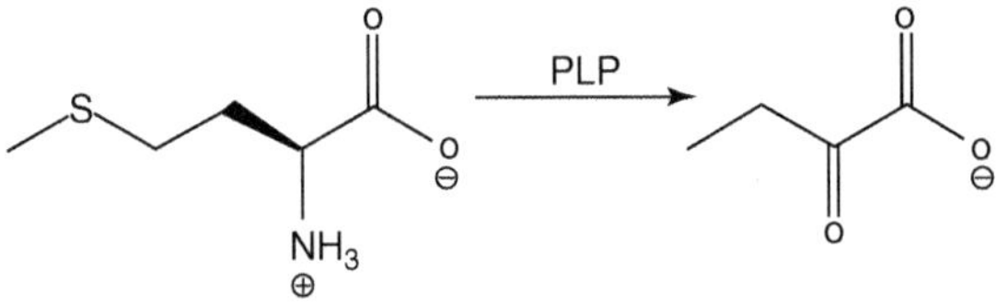

Fig. 5.6 Enzymatic activity of methionine γ-lyase

This negative charge may develop through (1) deprotonation of the alpha position, (2) decarboxylation of the amino acid, or (3) side-chain loss. Essentially one of the three groups at the < position is lost, leaving the bonding electron pair behind. This negative charge can then be resolved in one of the two ways: (1) by protonation or electrophile addition at the < position and subsequent hydrolysis or (2) by protonation at the imino-carbon of the pyridoxal, resulting in oxidation of the substrate and reduction of PLP to PAP. This is also outlined nicely on page 70 of the sourcebook.

® and © positions: Once a negative charge has developed, it may also be used for reaction at the ® position instead of resolution through protonation. There are two possibilities: (1) Elimination of a leaving group through an E1cb type mechanism; (2) deprotonation of the ® position and resolution by protonation of the imine nitrogen to affect further reactivity. Resolution by the second method often results in the expulsion of a leaving group at the © position. A classic example of this is the enzymatic activity of methionine ©-lyase, the action of which is schematized in Fig. 5.6.

Folic Acid and Vitamin B12: One Carbon Chemistry

Many reactions require the addition or removal of a single carbon from a molecule. These reactions generally require folic acid derivatives (or other molecules synthesized using folic acid derivatives, such as S-adenosylmethionine).

There are many folate derivatives with versatile functions in cellular biochemistry. N^5,N^{10}-methylene-tetrahydrofolate is essential in purine synthesis (several steps) and pyrimidine synthesis (thymidylate synthase) and for serine synthesis by serine hydroxymethyltransferase, all of which produce tetrahydrofolate as a byproduct. N^{10}-formyl-tetrahydrofolate is essential for purine synthesis. N^5-methyl-tetrahydrofolate is the primary form found in the diet and is required by methionine synthase. N^5-formimidoyltetrahydrofolate is used in histidine catabolism.

Index

A
Acetaminophen, 63
Acetoacetate, 48–50
Acetoacetyl-CoA, 49
Acetone, 48, 50
Acetyl-CoA, 22, 51, 108
Acetyl-CoA carboxylase, 51, 54
Acid hydrolases, 103
Activate PPARα, 82
Acute gout, 137
Acute intermittent porphyria, 119
Acyl-CoA, 42
Acyl-coA oxidase, 47
Acyl-CoA synthetase, 42, 56
Acyl-Coa:cholesterol acyltransferase (ACAT), 73
Acylglycerols, 56
Adenine phosphoribosyltransferase (APRT), 132
Adenosine deaminase deficiency, 134
Adenosine monophosphate, 128
Adrenocortical enzymes, 85
Adult respiratory distress syndrome (ARDS), 38
ALA dehydratase, 119
Alanine, 94
Alanine aminotransferase (ALT), 10, 94, 112
Alanine cycle, 112
Alanine transaminase (ALT), 105
Aldolase, 29
Aldolase A deficiency, 8
Alkaptonuria, 115, 123
Allantoin, 138
Allopurinol, 138
α-carbon, 91
α-keto decarboxylase complex, 118
α-Ketoglutarate dehydrogenase complex, 12
α-linolenic acid, 36
Amino acid degradation, 105
Amino acid metabolism, 93
  disease of, 122
  insulin and glucagon in, 118
  nutritionally nonessential amino acids, 93, 94, 96, 100
  nutritionally nonessential amino acids, 97
Aminosphingolipids, 41

Ammonia, 94
Ammonia transport, 111
Amphibolic pathway, 11
Analgesia, 67
Anandamide, 67
Androgens, 88
Antimycin A, 13
Apo AI, 77
Apo B-100, 75
Apo CII, 74
Apo E, 74
ApoB Editing Complex 1 (APOBEC1), 73
Apolipoproteins, 73
Arachidonic acid, 36, 63
Arginase, 108
Arginine, 100, 102, 108, 111
Arginine synthesis, 106, 108
Arginosuccinase (Arginosuccinate Lyase), 108
Arginosuccinate, 108
Arginosuccinate synthesis, 108
Arthritis, 115
Askhenazi Jews, 58
Asparagine, 94
Asparagine synthase, 94
Aspartate, 95, 108
Aspartate aminotransferase (AST), 95–96
Aspartate-arginosuccinate shunt, 106, 113
Aspirin, 13, 63
Atherogenesis, 77, 83
Atherosclerosis, 77, 89
Atorvastatin, 82
Autacoids, 62
Autophagy, 103

B

β-aminoisobutyrate, 142
β-D-glucose (β-D-glucopyranose), 2
β-galactosidases, 57
β-hydroxybutyrate, 48
β-hydroxybutyrate dehydrogenase, 48
β-oxidation, 44
Bile, 122
Bile acid resins, 82
Bile acids, 84
Bilirubin, 122
Biliverdin, 122
Biotin, 45
Block enterohepatic circulation, 82
Branched-chain amino acids, 117

C

Cannabinoids, 67
Carbamoyl phosphate, 106, 107, 139, 140
Carbamoyl phosphate synthase I (CPSI), 106
Carbamoyl phosphate synthase II (CPSII), 139
Carbamoyl phosphate synthesis, 106
Carbohydrate metabolism, 3
  enzyme deficiencies in, 34
  glycolysis, 4–9
  metabolic diseases, 33
  mitochondrial shuttles of, 14, 15
Carbon skeletons,
  catabolism of, 113
Cardiolipins, 39
Carnitine acylcarnitine translocase, 44
Carnitine deficiencies, 44
Carnitine palmitoyltransferase I (CPTI), 44, 55
Carnitine palmitoyl-transferase II, 44
Carnitine shuttle, 42–44
Catechol-O-methyltransferase (COMT), 102
CDP-choline, 56
CDP-ethanolamine, 56
Ceramidases, 57
Cerebrohepatorenal syndrome, 48

Chemiosmotic theory, 13
Chocolate cyanosis, 121
Cholesterol, 69, 73
Cholesterol absorption inhibitors, 82
Cholesterol biosynthesis, 70
Cholesterol ester transfer protein (CETP), 78
Cholesterol homeostasis, 83
Cholesterol metabolism, 84
Cholesteryl esters, 73, 78
Choline, 56, 96
Chronic gout, 138
Chylomicron, 74
Chylomicron remnants, 74, 78
Chylomicrons, 73–75
Cisterna chyli, 74
Citrate lyase, 51
Citrate shuttle, 51
Citric acid cycle, 11
Citrulline, 107, 108
Citrulline synthesis, 107
CoA transferase, 49
Cognitive deficits, 133
Colchicine, 138
Competitive inhibitors, 82
Complex lipids, 38
Congenital adrenal hyperplasia, 87
Congenital methemoglobinemia, 121
Conjugate addition, 151
Cori cycle, 24
COX-1, 63, 68
COX-2, 63, 68
COX-2 selective inhibition, 68
Creatine, 102
Crigler-Najjar syndrome, 122
Cystathionine β-synthase, 97
Cysteine, 97, 115
Cysteinyl leukotrienes, 66
Cystine kidney stone, 115
Cystine reductase, 115
Cystinuria, 115
Cytosol, 108
Cytosolic acetyl-CoA, 70
Cytosolic creatine, 16

Cytosolic fatty acid synthesis, 53

D

de novo synthesis, 136
Death from liver failure, 115
Deoxyribonucleotides, 126, 133
Desaturases, 54
Desmolase deficiency, 87
Diabetes mellitus, 72
Diabetic ketoacidosis, 49, 89
Diacylglycerol acyltransferase (DGAT), 56, 73
Dietary purines, 136
Dihydrobiopterin reductase, 100
Dihydrobiopterin synthase, 100
Dihydrofolate reductase, 131, 141
Dihydroorotate dehydrogenase, 141
Dihydroxyacetone phosphate (DHAP), 14
1, 25-dihydroxyvitamin D_3 (calcitriol), 89
Dipalmitoyl lecithin, 38
Disorders of Lipid Transport, 90
D-Methylmalonyl-CoA, 45
Docosahexaenoic acid (DHA), 37, 66, 67
Dopamine, 100
Dubin-Johnson syndrome, 122

E

Eczema, 99
Eicosanoid families, 67
Eicosanoids, 62, 63
Eicosapentaenoic acid (EPA), 37, 66, 67
Electron sink, 152
E1 ligase, 103
E2 ligase, 103
E3 ligase, 103
Encephalopathy, 46, 109
Endocannabinoid, 67
Endogenous hepatic cholesterol synthesis, 82

Endoplasmic reticulum, 53
Energetic matching, 150
Enzyme deficiencies in carbohydrate metabolism, 90
Epinephrine, 55, 100
Epoxins, 66
Ergocalciferol, 89
Essential amino acid, 99
Essential fatty acids, 36
Essential fructosuria, 29
Estradiol, 88
Even chain fatty acid, 46
Exercise, biochemical changes, 32, 33
Ezetimibe, 82

F

Fabry disease, 62
FAD/FADH$_2$ reductions, 151
Fasting hypoketotic hypoglycemia, 44, 90
Fats/oils, 37
Fatty acid degradation, 42
Fatty acid elongation, 53
Fatty acid synthesis, 51, 53
 and oxidation, 55
 regulation of, 54
Fatty acids, 35
 degradation, 42
 elongation, 53
 oxidation of, 42, 44–47
Female sex hormones, 88
Ferrochelatase, 119
Fibrates, 82
First committed step, 129
5-fluorouracil (5-FU), 141
Foam cells, 76
Folic acid, 96, 131, 155
Formyl transferase, 131
Fructokinase, 29
Fructose, 2
Fructose intolerance, 29
Fructose metabolism, 29

Fructose-1,6-bisphosphatase, 24
Fructose-2,6-bisphosphate (F2,6BP), 7
Fumarate, 108

G

Galactokinase, 31
Galactokinase deficiency, 31, 32
Galactose, 3
Galactose metabolism, 31
Galactose-1-phosphate uridyltransferase, 31
Galactosemia, 31, 32
Galactosylceramide, 41
γ-aminobutyric acid (GABA), 101
Gangliosides, 41, 57
Gaucher disease, 61
Gene therapy, 134
Gilbert syndrome, 122
Glectrochemical gradient, 13
Globoid cells, 61
Glucagon, 27, 55
 in amino acid metabolism, 118
Glucocorticoids, 138
Glucogenic amino acids, 113
Gluconeogenesis, 22
 fructose-1,6-bisphosphate to fructose-6-phosphate, 24
 glucose-6-phosphate to glucose, 24
 pyruvate to phosphoenol pyruvate, 22
Glucose, 2
Glucose metabolism, 27
Glucose, phosphorylation of, 5
Glucose-1-phosphate, 17
Glucose-6-phosphatase, 20, 24
Glucose-6-phosphate, 6
Glucose-6-phosphate dehydrogenase (G6PD) deficiency, 27
Glucuronic acid, 122
Glutamate, 94, 97, 101, 105, 108
Glutamate decarboxylase, 101–102

Glutamate dehydrogenase, 94, 106
Glutamate synthase, 94
Glutamate-derived neurotransmitters, 101
Glutaminase, 106, 111
Glutamine, 94, 105
Glutamine cycle, 111
Glutamine synthase, 94, 111
Glycerol phosphate shuttle, 9, 14
Glycerol-3-phosphate dehydrogenase, 56
Glycerolipids metabolism, 56
Glycerolphosphate shuttle, 14
Glycerophospholipids, 38
Glycine, 96, 102, 113
Glycogen, 2, 16
Glycogen storage disorders (GSD), 21, 22
Glycogen synthesis, 16, 18
Glycogenolysis, 19–21
Glycolipids, 40, 57
Glycolysis
  ATP through the dephosphorylation of 1,3-bisphosphoglycerate, 8
  dehydrates 2-phosphoglycerate, 9
  isomerization of dihydroxyacetone phosphate to glyceraldehyde phosphate, 8
  isomerization of glucose-6-phosphate to fructose-6-phosphate, 6
  isomerization of phosphoglycerate, 9
  NADH through the oxidative-phosphorylation of GAP, 8
  phosphorylation of fructose-6-phosphate, 7
  phosphorylation of glucose, 5
  pyruvate, 9
  reverse aldol (retroaldol) cleavage, 8
Glycosphingolipids, 40

Glyoxylate reductase/hydroxypyruvate reductase (GRHPR), 113
Gout
  lifestyle management, 137
  pathophysiology and clinical manifestations, 137
  phases, 137
Guanosine monophosphate, 128

H

Half-reaction, 149
Harmful Fats, 37
Hemoglobin, 121
Hepatic encephalopathy, 109, 122
Hepatic lipase, 76
Hepatic scavenger receptors, 79
Hexokinase, 5, 6
Hexosaminidases, 57
Hexose monophosphate shunt, 25, 27
Hexoses, 2
Histamine, 100
HMG-CoA reductase, 82
HMG-CoA reductase, regulation of, 72
HMG-CoA synthase, 48, 70
Homocitrullinuria syndrome (HHH), 110
Homocysteine, 98
Homocysteinuria, 98, 122
Homogentisate oxidase, 115
Hormone, 84
Hormone sensitive lipase, 55
Hunter syndrome, 62
Hurler syndrome, 62
3-hydroxybutyrate, 48
3-hydroxybutyrate dehydrogenase, 48
1-α-hydroxylase, 89
7α-hydroxylase, 84
25-hydroxylase, 89
17α-hydroxylase deficiency, 87
21-hydroxylase deficiency, 87

3β-hydroxysteroid dehydrogenase deficiency, 87
5-hydroxytryptamine, 5-HT, 100
Hyperammonemia, 110
Hyperammonemia type I, 110
Hyperammonemia type II, 110
Hyperglycemia, 31, 49
Hyperornithinemia, 110
Hyperprolinemias, 117
Hyperuricemia, 136
    dietary causes, 136
    excretory causes, 136
Hypoxanthine guanine phosphoribosyl transferase (HGPRT) deficiency, 132, 136

I

IMP dehydrogenase, 131
Inborn errors of metabolism, 136
Inosine monophosphate (IMP), 128, 129
Insulin
    in amino acid metabolism, 118
Insulin action in muscle or fat, 27
Insulin action in the liver, 28
Insulin and exercise, 32
Insulin in fatty acid metabolism, 54
Insulin synthesis, 27
Interesterified fat, 38
Intermittent branched-chain ketonuria, 118
Inulin, 2
Ionophores (uncouplers), 13
Isoleucine, 113
Isoprostanes, 66, 67
Isovaleric acidemia, 118

K

Ketoacidosis, 50
Ketogenesis, 69

Ketogenic amino acids, 113
Ketone body formation, 48
Kidney, 89
Krabbe disease, 61
Kreb's cycle, 11
Kwashiorkor, 92

L

L-amino acids, 91
Lanosterol, 70
LDL receptor, 74
LDL-receptor related protein (LRP), 74
Lecithin:cholesterol acyltransferase (LCAT), 78
Lefluno mide, 141
Lesch-Nyhan syndrome, 132, 136
Leucine, 113
Leukotriene B_4 (LTB$_4$), 66
Leukotrienes, 66
Limit phenylalanine intake, 99
Linoleic acid, 36
Lipid metabolism
    cholesterol biosynthesis, 70
    cholesterol homeostasis, 83
    COX-2 selective inhibition, 68
    disease of, 89
    eicosanoids, 63, 66, 67
    fatty acid elongation, 53
    HMG-CoA reductase, regulation of, 72
    insulin in fatty acid metabolism, 54
    lipid transport, 73, 74, 76, 78
    lipogenesis, 51
    metabolic changes during fasting, 68
    monounsaturated and polyunsaturated fatty acids, 54
    oxidation of fatty acids, 42, 44–47
    oxidation of unsaturated fatty acids, 47

sphingolipidoses and sulfatidoses, 58
sphingolipids metabolism, 57
Lipid transport, 72, 75
  disorders of, 79, 82
Lipid-lowering drugs, 82
Lipogenesis, 51
Lipoprotein (a), 79
Lipoprotein lipase (LPL), 74
Lipoprotein X, 79
Lipoproteins, 73, 79
Lipoxins, 66
Lipoxygenase pathway, 66
Liver, 89
Lovastatin, 82
Low alcohol diet, 136
Low-density lipoproteins (LDL), 76
Lymphatics, 74
Lysine, 103, 113
Lysosomal degradation, 103

M

Macrophages, 122
Malate shuttle, 9, 14
Malate-aspartate shuttle, 9, 14
Malonyl-CoA, 51, 55
Maple syrup urine disease, 117–118
Marasmus, 92, 122
Matched redox reactions, 150
Maturity onset diabetes of the young (MODY), 28, 34
Medium chain acyl-CoA dehydrogenase (MCAD), 44
Melanin, 102
Melatonin, 100
Metabolic changes during fasting, 68
Metabolic syndrome, 28
Metformin, 32, 33
Methemoglobinemia, 121
Methionine, 97, 115
Methionine synthase, 97
Methotrexate, 131, 141
Methylene blue, 121
Methylmalonic acidemia, 46

Methylmalonyl-CoA isomerase, 45, 46
Methylmalonyl-CoA mutase, 46
Microsomal fatty acid elongase system, 53
Microsomal heme oxygenase system, 122
Microsomal system, 54
Microsomal transfer protein, 74
Mitochondrial fatty acid oxidation, 47
Mitochondrial matrix, 107
Mitochondrial shuttle, 9
Molecular O_2, 84
Monosaccharides, 1
Monounsaturated fatty acids, 35, 37, 54
Motor dysfunction, 133
Multiple sclerosis, 39
Musty odor, 99
Mycophenolic acid, 131
Myelin formation, 53

N

N-acetylglutamate, 108
N-acetylglutamate synthase, 108–109
NADH-cytochrome b_5 reductase, 121
Nascent HDL particle, 77
Neuraminidic acid, 57
Neurotransmitters, 100
Nicotinamide adenine dinucleotide (NAD), 151
Niemann-Pick disease, 61
Nitric oxide, 102
Nitric oxide synthase (NOS), 102
Norepinephrine, 100
NPC1L1, 73
Nucleoside kinase, 140, 142
Nucleoside phosphorylase, 140, 141
Nucleotide metabolism
  de novo purine biosynthesis, 130
  deoxyribonucleotides synthesis, 133

disease of, 143
purine nucleotide biosynthesis, 127
purine salvage, 131
pyrimidine biosynthesis, 138
urate pools, 136
uric acid production, 134
Nucleotides, biologically important, 125–127
Nutrasweet, 99
Nutritionally essential amino acids, 91
Nutritionally nonessential amino acids, 92–94, 96, 97, 100

O

Obesity, 28, 34
Ochronosis, 115
Oligomycin, 13
Ornithine, 107, 108
Ornithine transcarbamoylase, 107
Ornithine transporter, 108
Orotic aciduria, 140
Osteomalacia, 89
Oxaloacetate, 46
Oxidation half-reaction, 149
Oxidation of fatty acids, 42, 44–47
Oxidation of unsaturated fatty acids, 47
Oxidative phosphorylation, 12, 13
Oxidative stress, 66
Oxidizing agent, 149

P

Painful abdomen, 119
Palmitic acid, 35, 51, 53
Pan-metabolic diseases, 72
Partial hydrogenation, 37
Pentose phosphate pathway, 25, 27
Peroxins, 48
Peroxisomal fatty acid metabolism, 47
Peroxisomal fatty acid oxidation, 47
Phenylacetate, 110
Phenylalanine, 99, 113, 115
Phenylalanine hydroxylase, 99, 115
Phenylketonuria, 99, 122
Phosphate, 128
Phosphatidalcholine, 39
Phosphatidalethanolamine, 39
Phosphatidate, 56
Phosphatidate phosphohydrolase, 56
Phosphatidic acid (phosphatidate), 38, 56
Phosphatidylcholines (lecithins), 38
Phosphatidylethanolamines, 38
Phosphatidylinositols, 39
Phosphatidylserines, 39
Phosphodiester bonds, 126
Phosphoenol pyruvate, 22
Phosphoenolpyruvate carboxykinase, 22
Phosphofructokinase-1, 6
Phosphofructokinase-2, 7
Phosphoglucomutase, 17
3-phosphoglycerate, 96
Phospholipase A_2, 63
Phospholipases, 57, 67
Phospholipids, 38
Phosphoribosyl pyrophosphate (PRPP), 128
Phosphoribosylamine, 128, 129
Phosphorylation of fructose-6-phosphate, 7
Phosphorylation of glucose, 5
Photosensitivity, 119
Pink urine, 119
Plasmalogens, 39
Pleasure sensing pathways, 67
Polyneuropathy, 119
Polysaccharides, 2
Polyubiquitinated, Ubiquitin, 103
Polyunsaturated fatty acids, 35, 37, 54
Porphyria cutanea tarda, 119
Porphyrias, 118
Porphyrin, 102
Porphyrin degradation, 122

Porphyrin synthesis, 118
Potential gradient, 150
Pravastatin, 82
Primary hyperoxaluria, 113
Probenecid, 138
Progesterone, 88
Proline, 97, 117
Propionic acidemia, 46
Propionyl-CoA carboxylase, 45, 46
Prostacyclins, 66
Prostaglandin E_2 (PGE_2), 66
Prostaglandins, 63
Prostanoids, 63
Proteases, 103
Proteasomal degradation, 103
Proteasome, 103
Protectins, 66
Protein degradation, 103
Protein synthesis, 102
Protonated amine, 91
PRPP glutamyl amidotransferase, 128, 131
PRPP synthase, 128
Psychological disturbances, 119
Purine degradation, 134
Purine nucleotide biosynthesis, 127–129
Purine salvage, 131
Purine synthesis enzymes, chemotherapeutic agents for block, 131
Pyridoxal phosphate (PLP), 95, 96, 102, 106, 152
Pyridoxine, 152
Pyrimidine biosynthesis, 139
Pyrimidine biosynthesis, regulation of, 140
Pyrimidine degradation, 142
Pyrimidine salvage, 141
Pyrimidine synthesis enzymes, chemotherapeutic agents that block, 141
Pyrophosphatase, 17
Pyrophosphate (PPi), 17
Pyruvate, 9, 22
Pyruvate carboxylase, 22
Pyruvate dehydrogenase, 10
Pyruvate metabolism, 9, 10

R

Rasburicase, 138
Rate determining step, 129
Rate limiting step, 101, 106
Rational drug design, 142
REDOX chemistry, 149
Redox reactions, 151
Reducing agent, 149
Reduction half-reaction, 149
Reduction-oxidation (Redox), 149
Resolvins, 66
Reticuloendothelial system, 122
Retinitis pigmentosa, 37
Reverse Aldol (Retroaldol) cleavage, 8
Reverse cholesterol transport, 74, 75, 77
Ribonucleotide reductase, 133
Ribonucleotides, 125
Ribose, 25
Ribose-5'-monophosphate, 128
Richner-Hanhart syndrome, 115
Rosuvastatin, 82
Rotenone, 13
Rotor syndrome, 122

S

S-Adenosylmethionine (SAM), 100
Salt retention, 87
Salt wasting, 87
Salvage-gene therapy, 136
Saturated fatty acids, 35, 37
Scavenger receptors, 76
Serine, 96, 97
Serine hydroxymethyltransferase, 96
Serotonin (5-hydroxytryptamine, 5-HT), 100
Serum glutamate oxaloacetate transaminase (SGOT), 96

Serum glutamate pyruvate transaminase (SGPT), 94–95
Severe combined immunodeficiency (SCID), 134
Severe disfigurement, 119
Severe mental disorders, 46
Simple Lipids, 37
Simvastatin, 82
Sodium benzoate, 110
Sorbitol pathway, 31
Sphingolipases, 57
Sphingolipidoses, 57, 58
Sphingolipids, 40
Sphingolipids metabolism, 57
Sphingomyelins, 40, 57
Statins, 72, 82
Steroids, 84, 85
Sterol regulatory element binding protein (SREBP), 72
Succinate Thiokinase, 12
Succinyl-CoA, 46
Sulfatidoses, 58
Sulfosphingolipids, 41
Supplement tyrosine, 99

T

Taurine, 102
Tay-Sachs disease, 58
Testosterone, 88
Tetrahydrobiopterin, 99
Tetrahydrofolate, 140
Thermogenin (UCP1), 13
Thiolase, 70
Thiophorase, 49
Thioredoxin, 133
Thoracic duct, 74
Thromboxanes, 66
Thymidylate synthase, 140, 141
Thyroxine (thyroid hormone), 100
Tissue paper macrophages, 61
Torcetrapib, 82
Transaminases, 105
Transamination, 95, 105
Triacylglycerols, 56
Tryptophan, 113
Tryptophan hydroxylation, 100

Tryptophan-derived neurotransmitters, 100
Type 1 diabetes mellitus, 28, 33
Type 2 diabetes mellitus, 28, 33
Tyrosine, 99, 102, 113, 115
Tyrosine hydroxylase, 100
Tyrosine-derived neurotransmitters, 100
Tyrosines, 100

U

Ubiquitin activating protein, 103
Ubiquitin ligase, 103
Ubiquitin transfer protein, 103
Unsaturated fatty acids oxidation of, 47
Urate, 132, 134
Urate Pools, 136
Urea, 108
Urea cycle, 100, 106
  arginine synthesis, 106, 108
  arginosuccinate synthesis, 108
  carbamoyl phosphate synthesis, 106
  citrulline synthesis, 107
  defects, 110
  for elimination of nitrogenous wastes, 106
  regulation of, 108
  urea synthesis, 108
Urea synthesis, 108
Uric acid, 132, 134
Uricase, 138
Uridine diphosphogalactose-4 epimerase, 31
Uridine monophosphate (UMP) synthase, 140
Urinary reabsorption, 136

V

Very high dose niacin, 82
Very long chain fatty acids (VLCFAs), 47
Virilization, 87
Vitamin B_6, 152

Vitamin B$_6$
    (pyridoxine), 93, 95, 96, 106
Vitamin B$_{12}$, 155
Vitamin C, 84
Vitamin D biosynthesis, 88
Vitamin D deficiency, 89
Vitamins, REDOX
    Chemistry, 149

W
Waxes, 38

X
Xanthine oxidase, 134, 138
Xanthine oxidase
    inhibitors, 136
X-linked adrenoleukodystrophy, 47

Z
Zellweger syndrome, 48
Zwitterion, 91